George M Sternberg

Supply table of the Medical Department, United States Army,

1894

George M Sternberg

Supply table of the Medical Department, United States Army, 1894

ISBN/EAN: 9783742818485

Manufactured in Europe, USA, Canada, Australia, Japa

Cover: Foto ©Lupo / pixelio.de

Manufactured and distributed by brebook publishing software
(www.brebook.com)

George M Sternberg

Supply table of the Medical Department, United States Army,

1894

SUPPLY TABLE

OF THE

MEDICAL DEPARTMENT,

UNITED STATES ARMY.

1894.

WAR DEPARTMENT,
SURGEON GENERAL'S OFFICE,
WASHINGTON, *April 25, 1894.*

The following is the Supply Table of the Medical Department of the United States Army, and its provisions and requirements will be in force from this date.

GEO. M. STERNBERG,

Surgeon General, U. S. Army.

Approved :

DANIEL S. LAMONT,

Secretary of War.

WAR DEPARTMENT, *April 26, 1894.*

SUPPLY TABLE.

1. The Supply Table enumerates the medical supplies issued to the U. S. Army, and the quantities and sizes of original packages.

It is the policy of the Medical Department to supply, from time to time, new remedies of determined therapeutic value ; but newly introduced remedies desired only for experiment and such as offer no manifest advantage over those already issued will not be supplied. It should be borne in mind that these supplies are selected for *the military service.* It is believed that all necessary articles are included and that the quantities allowed will be found sufficient under ordinary circumstances.

Requisitions for particular preparations simply because they are agreeable to the taste, or to save trouble in compounding, will not be approved ; nor will preparations of a drug be furnished when one or more practically equivalent ones are on the list.

2. The senior medical officer of every post will make annual requisitions for medical supplies for the year commencing January first, unless another date is fixed by the Surgeon General. Such requisitions will be made in triplicate and forwarded to the medical director, or, in the case of independent posts, in duplicate, to the Surgeon General.

Medical directors will see that annual requisitions do not call for any article not on the Supply Table nor for quantities in excess of those therein allowed. They will forward one copy to the Surgeon General, one, with their approval, direct to the medical supply depot designated by the Surgeon General for issue, and will retain one in their office.

a. Annual requisitions will not be forwarded to the medical director more than twenty days before the date at which the period they cover begins. They will be made only for articles that are, or probably will be, needed during the year, will state the quantity of all articles on hand, *as verified by a medical officer* in accordance with par. 18 b, and will give the total number of persons entitled

by regulations to medicines. Quantities on hand will be
deducted from the quantities allowed by the Supply Table.

b. Medical directors at their inspections will carefully
investigate the method of preparing requisitions, particu-
larly as to the necessity for the quantities asked for and
the accuracy with which the amounts on hand are stated.

Supplies for tem-
porary posts, sub-
posts, and camps.

3. Requisitions for supplies for temporary posts or for
those soon to be abandoned will be confined to such articles as are absolutely necessary.

a. Subposts and camps will, in absence of orders to
the contrary, obtain such medical supplies as may be
required by requisition upon the senior medical officer
of the post to which they are subsidiary, who will issue
them after approval by the medical director.

All articles not
issued to smaller
posts.

4. It is not expected that the smaller posts will require
for all the articles included in these lists, and the local
prevalence or rarity of certain diseases, as well as the
quantity or number on hand of each article, will be considered in the preparation and approval of requisitions.

Special requisi-
tions.

5. When medical supplies are absolutely necessary
before the annual requisition is prepared they should
be required for upon a special requisition, in triplicate,
giving a list of the articles needed, and the quantity on
hand, and giving explicit reasons for the necessity of
such requisition. These will be transmitted through the
medical director, who will retain one copy and will forward two to the Surgeon General.

Medical directors will personally and carefully scruti-
nize the requisitions, and make such changes therein as
they may deem proper.

a. The quantities asked for will be computed on the
basis of original packages.

b. Proper care in the preparation of the annual requisition should prevent the necessity of requiring for any-
thing but medicines and hospital stores on special requisitions, and the necessity for an additional supply of
these should be rare.

c. Special requisitions for instruments, books, bedding,
furniture, etc., will seldom be approved.

Nomenclature,
etc., to be followed.

6. In all returns, requisitions, invoices, and receipts
pertaining to medical supplies, the nomenclature, order
of entry, and classification of the Supply Table will be
strictly followed, and the copies will be carefully com-
pared.

a. They will be forwarded without letters of transmittal.

7. While it is believed that the quantities of medicines and hospital stores allowed will be ample and usually in excess of the requirements, it is not supposed that they will always meet the necessities caused by the prevalence of epidemics or by the location of troops in unhealthy parts of the country. Medical officers who allow their supplies to become exhausted in such contingencies without giving timely notice of the deficiency will be held accountable for any bad results arising therefrom. *Medical officers responsible for ample supplies.*

8. In cases of emergency, as sudden epidemics, not admitting of delay, medical directors are authorized to act upon special requisitions, forwarding one copy, with their action, to the nearest medical supply depot, one to the Surgeon General, with an indorsement stating the circumstances, and retaining one; but requisitions for articles not on the Supply Table must, in all cases, be forwarded to the Surgeon General for his action. *Requisitions to meet emergencies.*

9. Officers in charge of medical supply depots will not issue any article not on this Supply Table, except by special authority of the Surgeon General. *Articles not on Supply Table issued only by authority of Surgeon General.*

10. In view of the present universal telegraphic facilities between posts and Department headquarters and Washington, D. C., the authority given in A. R. 1648 is revoked. *Authority to purchase medicines in emergency revoked.*

11. Officers transferring medical supplies will prepare invoices (Form No. 21) in duplicate, one for the Surgeon General and one for the receiving officer. The receiving officer will prepare receipts (Form No. 23) in duplicate, one for the Surgeon General, with a report of the condition of the articles, and one for the issuing officer. The vouchers for the Surgeon General will be promptly forwarded after the transfer is completed. A packer's list (Form No. 20) will, if necessary, be furnished by the issuing officer. *Transfer of medical supplies.*

12. On assuming charge of medical property great care should be exercised before receipting for cases of instruments, microscopes, and other property of similar character not enumerated on the property papers in detail, to ascertain that the full contents of such cases are present and in good order. Incomplete cases will be so receipted for, and a list of the missing instruments, etc., will accompany the receipt in order that the proper officer may be held accountable for the deficiency. *Receipts for property.*

a. Receipts, without remark, for cases of instruments and similar property will be considered as evidence that they are complete and in accordance with the lists of contents given in this Supply Table, and the receiving officer will thereafter be held responsible in accordance therewith.

b. The issuing officer will enter on his invoices, and the receiving officer on his receipts, the condition of all articles not serviceable.

Condition of property received.

13. Medical officers will report to the Surgeon General, and to the issuing officer all defects observed in the quality, quantity, or packing of medical supplies. They are requested to freely communicate to the Surgeon General any suggestions tending to the improvement of medical supplies, appliances, etc., and to make reports as to new designs of apparatus, field equipment, etc.

Loss or destruction of non-expendable articles.

14. When non-expendable articles are lost or destroyed the circumstances of the loss or destruction must be fully set forth in a certificate from the officer responsible for the property, or in a certificate of a commissioned officer cognizant of the facts, or, in the absence of these, in an affidavit of a non-interested person. If the evidence is considered satisfactory by the Surgeon General, the responsible officer will be so informed and authorized to drop the articles from his returns. If not satisfactory he will be required to replace them at his own expense.

Expendable and non-expendable articles indicated.

15. The names of all expendable articles are printed in Roman type ; those of all non-expendable articles are in Italics.

Supplies to be taken up.

16. Medical officers will take up and account for all medical supplies of the Army that come into their possession, and report, when possible, to whose account they are to be credited.

Medical property needing repair.

17. Surgical instruments and appliances that require and are considered worth repairing will be reported to the Surgeon General through the medical director, with a statement of the repairs needed.

a. When requisition is made to complete a broken or imperfect instrument or apparatus, the name of the maker will be given. Instruments of different makes have been issued, and such information is required to insure the proper pattern and fit of the parts asked for.

Care of property.

18. Medical officers will be held directly responsible for the serviceable and complete condition of all property in their possession except such as may have been rendered unserviceable by fair wear and tear.

a. The responsible officer will cause all instruments in his charge to be examined by a commissioned medical officer at least once each month.

b. He will also twice each year cause all medical property in his charge to be carefully examined by a commissioned medical officer, and verified by the returns, invoices, etc.

19. Medical officers will submit to the medical director at his annual inspection such articles of furniture as chairs, bedside tables, and property of that general class which may need and are considered worth repair or renovation by painting, varnishing, etc. This should be done by post labor, if practicable, request being made to the Surgeon General for authority to purchase necessary material. If not practicable, the medical officer will obtain one or more estimates in detail of cost of repair or renovation of such furniture, etc., as may be designated by the medical director, and forward them through the medical director for the action of the Surgeon General. *Repair of furniture.*

20. Medical officers in charge of medical supplies will prepare annually, on December 31, unless another date is fixed by the Surgeon General, or when relieved from the charge thereof, returns of medical supplies (Form No. 25) in duplicate, showing those on hand at last return, those received, expended, issued, and sold, and those remaining on hand. *Property returns of medical officers.*

a. The original of this return will be promptly transmitted to the Surgeon General. The duplicate, with a complete set of vouchers, will be retained for the protection of the officer responsible for the property.

b. In exceptional cases a certified invoice may be offered by the issuing officer, in the absence of a receipt, as a substitute for the proper voucher, together with such additional evidence as he may possess in regard to the transfer.

c. No interlineations or erasures will be made on the returns, and all articles not provided for in the printed headings will be entered in proper order under the heading of additional articles.

21. Articles issued to posts shall not be taken away by the medical officer on being relieved, nor when absent on leave, except by authority of the Surgeon General or of a medical director. *Post medical property not to be taken away.*

22. Damaged and unserviceable medical property will not be presented to an inspector for condemnation until authority for so doing has been obtained from the Surgeon General. *Inspection of damaged and unserviceable medical property.*

a. At independent posts and supply depots recommendations relating to unserviceable property will be made by the officer responsible for the same, or by a medical officer detailed for the purpose; at other posts by the medical director of the department.

b. Lists of unserviceable articles (Form No. 43) will be prepared in duplicate, and the property submitted to the medical director upon his annual visit to the post.

c. Medical directors, when they have personally inspected medical property thus submitted to them, may authorize the officer accountable for the same to submit such portion as in their opinion is proper to an officer of the Inspector General's Department, with a view to condemnation, by the following indorsement: "To be submitted for the action of an inspector. By authority of the Surgeon General. (Signed) ——— ———." In this case one copy will be left with the officer accountable for the property and one will be forwarded at once to the Surgeon General.

d. If circumstances should require an inspection of unserviceable property at other times, this list, in duplicate, will be forwarded through the medical director to the Surgeon General, who will give instructions as to the disposition of the property.

Sale of medical property.

23. When condemned medical property is sold at public auction the officer responsible therefor will prepare an account of sales (Form No. 12) in duplicate. He will also prepare an invoice (Form No. 13) in duplicate of the articles sold. The original of this account of sales, accompanied by the original invoice and a copy of the inventory and inspection report, will be sent at once to the Surgeon General; the duplicate copies of each will be filed by the officer with his retained set of vouchers.

Proceeds of sale.

24. Medical officers receiving money from the sale of public property will deposit the same, without delay, in the nearest Government depository to the credit of the Treasurer of the United States, taking duplicate certificates of deposit therefor, the original of which will be forwarded by the depositor, without letter of transmittal, direct to the Secretary of the Treasury, Washington, D. C., and the duplicate retained by him. Should it be necessary to incur any expenses in connection with such sales they will be paid out of the total receipts before depositing the latter, in which case the expenses will be supported by properly prepared and receipted vouchers attached to the account of sales.

25. Medical officers in charge of medical property will not permit it to be used for other than hospital purposes. Medical directors will report every instance in which this regulation is violated. Medical property not to be used for other than hospital purposes.

a. This regulation, however, is not to be construed as prohibiting medical officers from using such medical property as books, instruments, etc., wherever they may deem necessary.

b. Under no circumstances will hospital bedding be used except within the hospital to which it has been supplied, nor will it be used by members of the hospital corps except when on duty in the wards.

26. Hospital clothing shall be worn by patients only during their stay in hospital. Each article will be marked as medical property. When very sick soldiers are transferred from one hospital to another the hospital clothing necessary for their comfort may be sent with them, properly invoiced, and accompanied by a check list giving the names of the men in whose possession it is. Use of hospital clothing.

a. Crutches and similar articles may, if necessary, be similarly transferred with the patient from one post or hospital to another under the provisions of this paragraph.

27. Medicines may be dispensed to persons entitled to medical attendance, and hospital stores to enlisted men and hospital matrons; also to officers at posts or stations where they can not be procured by purchase. Issue of medicines and hospital stores.

a. The regulation that officers and others are not entitled to any articles on the list of hospital stores if such can be obtained at or near their station will be strictly complied with.

b. Hospital matrons are not entitled to hospital stores except when prescribed for them as patients; the regulation is not to be construed as authorizing the issue to them of soap or lye for laundry use.

c. The issue of articles for use in the preparation of cleaning mixtures, cosmetics, perfumery, use with spirit lamps, etc., is strictly prohibited.

28. The exchange of medicines with druggists is prohibited. Exchange of medicines prohibited.

29. There is no authority of law or regulation for the sale or supply of medicines to civilians not employés of the Army, except as patients in hospital. If a medical officer assumes the responsibility of issuing medicines to sick civilians he must comply with the letter and spirit of the decision of the Secretary of War as promulgated Sale of medicines.

in Par. IV, Circular 10, A. G. O., 1890, in justification of his action.

Care of blankets. 30. Blankets not in use should be frequently examined and occasionally shaken and hung out of doors. When stained and soiled, but otherwise in good condition, they should be washed and continued in service. When deemed necessary, authority will be given to have them washed at a steam laundry if one is near the post.

Sectional mattresses. 31. When the present supply of hair mattresses is exhausted the "sectional" mattress in three parts will be issued. Three sections constitute a mattress, but as the end pieces will be serviceable much longer than the middle one, the latter may be inspected and condemned as mattress ⅓, and the others carried on the returns as mattress ⅔, etc.

Laundry accessories. 32. Laundry appliances will no longer be supplied to post hospitals. Washtubs will be furnished for the purpose of soaking sheets, clothing, etc., in disinfecting solutions.

Vaccine virus. 33. Requests for vaccine virus should be made direct to the Surgeon General by information slip. On account of its liability to become inert from various causes, especially from heat, it should be asked for in such quantities only as are needed for early use. It will hereafter be supplied only in the form of non-humanized (bovine) virus on charged points, ten points in each package.

Disinfectants. 34. Disinfectants are issued, as are medicines, to be used by medical officers when actually required for some specific purpose. The routine giving out of disinfectants to be scattered about the post is prohibited, and medical directors will, at their inspections, carefully investigate the use of these articles.

The requirements of circular from this office of August 9, 1893, will be strictly complied with.

Antiseptic dressings. 35. Sterilized dressings will not be issued for post use. Their preparation is so simple and so well understood that they should be prepared as needed. First-aid packets will be reserved exclusively for field use, except as occasionally needed for the instruction of members of the hospital corps.

Pens. 36. Pens of four common and generally used patterns will be issued as required, namely: falcon, stub, large fine, and small fine.

Use of field furniture. 37. Field furniture will not be used at posts except when required for the instruction of men of the hospital corps.

38. Medical and surgical chests will be frequently *Medical and surgical chests.* inspected and kept in perfect order for immediate field use. Under no circumstances will their contents be used at posts.

39. Pieces of canvas of the proper size for litters will *Canvas for litters.* be issued as required to replace pieces that may be torn or unserviceable. If soiled, the canvas should be removed from the litter, washed, and replaced.

40. Rubber and flexible catheters and bougies will be *Catheter box.* kept in the catheter box, using talc (French chalk) or glycerin to preserve them.

41. Field tourniquets and first-aid packets for the equip- *Field tourniquets and first-aid packets for company bearers.* ment of company bearers when serving in the field will be kept by the post surgeon until the necessity for such service arises. Before the departure of troops he will issue the required number to each company commander. taking his memorandum receipt therefor. Upon the return of the command the articles will be returned to the post surgeon. First-aid packets are expendable. If tourniquets thus issued are lost while in possession of a company commander, report of the fact should be made to the Surgeon General by the medical officer responsible, stating the circumstances of the loss, and requesting authority to drop the missing articles from his returns. If the command while in the field is ordered to another station, the post surgeon thereat will, upon its arrival, receive the tourniquets and packets, invoices and receipts being exchanged by the issuing and receiving officers.

42. Clinical thermometers are issued from the Surgeon *Clinical thermometers.* General's office upon request by information slip direct. giving number on hand and accompanied by a certificate of the medical officer in case of breakage, giving the name of the person who caused such loss and the number of the thermometer.

43. Record and copying ribbons for typewriting ma- *Typewriting accessories.* chines should be asked for by information slip as required, as they deteriorate if kept on hand any great length of time. Care should be exercised in the proper use of these ribbons for the purposes indicated by their names.

44. Meteorological instruments will not in future be *Meteorological instruments.* issued by the Medical Department. When required for use at designated posts they will be obtained by application direct to the Chief of the Weather Bureau, Department of Agriculture, Washington, D. C., specifying explicitly the kind of instruments required. When such instruments are broken or unserviceable the request for

a new one will contain a statement setting forth the circumstances attending the breakage, and the parts of the instrument, if a thermometer, will be returned to the office of the Weather Bureau by mail. Receipts for these instruments will be made out by the post surgeon on forms forwarded with the instruments, and when relieved from duty at the station he will so notify the Chief of the Weather Bureau, in order that the responsibility for the property may be properly transferred. Meteorological instruments heretofore issued by the Medical Department will be borne upon the property returns until broken or worn out. Such as may be issued by the Weather Bureau will not be taken up on these returns. The following will be issued: Maximum and minimum thermometers, rain and snow gauges, and measuring rods.

Ice machines.

45. Ice machines are issued to such southern posts as are unable to obtain by purchase ice for the use of the sick. They are furnished by the Medical Department to supply ice for the use of the sick in hospital, and not for the comfort or convenience of the garrison at large; but surplus ice may be sold in accordance with the provisions of Circular, S. G. O., June 13, 1891. They will be accounted for and invoiced in detail.

Individual equipment.

46. Emergency and field cases, hospital corps pouches, and similar articles of individual use or equipment, will be issued in accordance with the usual personnel of each hospital.

Screens and wire netting.

47. If window and door screens of unusual sizes are required, the requisition therefor should be accompanied by an estimate of cost of having suitable frames made at or near the post. Wire netting will be furnished to complete them and to renew such as have become unserviceable.

Bed screens.

48. When the present supply of bed screens is exhausted no more will be issued from depot. When required, application will be made to have the frames constructed at post, giving estimate of the cost; they will not in future be covered with holland, but sheets will be placed on the screens and frequently washed.

Prescriptions to be placed on file.

49. All prescriptions will be placed on file; those for liquors will be placed on a separate file.

Cocoa matting.

50. Cocoa matting in strips 1 meter wide is supplied for use on the floors of halls, and not for use on stairways or in wards. It should be laid in one strip, and zinc ends will be issued as required, two for each strip. It should not be nailed to the floor.

51. The expense of replating the silver-plated knives, forks, and spoons being about equal to their first cost, such articles will in future, when worn and unsuitable for table use, be submitted to the medical director for inspection, with a view to dropping them as originally issued and taking them up as "common" for kitchen use. Silver-plated cutlery.

52. Chemical and bacteriological sets will only be issued to the larger posts, and officers to whom these sets are furnished will be required to make an annual report on December 31, showing what use has been made of them. Issue of chemical and bacteriological sets.

53. Unless modified by special instructions from the Surgeon General, medical directors will be governed by the following general rules as to the disposition to be made of medical property upon the abandonment of a post: Dispo al of medical property upon abandonment of post.

(*a*.) Medicines, dressings, clothing, bedding, and miscellaneous articles in good and serviceable condition should be sent to other posts in the department.

(*b*.) Obsolete books which have been replaced by more modern ones and all unserviceable property should be submitted to the action of an inspector, with a view to final disposition by sale or destruction.

(*c*.) Only such non-expendable articles as are in perfect order, including recent medical works, and all instruments which can not be transferred to other posts without unnecessary duplication, should be turned into a medical supply depot.

54. No list of medical books is included in the present supply table, as, owing to the rapid advances in medicine, a large part of any fixed list soon becomes obsolete. Such new books as may be selected by the Surgeon General will be furnished without requisition. Medical books.

55. The library of the Surgeon General's office is intended for reference rather than circulation, but books that can be readily replaced will be loaned to medical officers of the Army, they being held responsible for the safe return of the volumes within two weeks from the day of their receipt. In special cases this time may be extended. Such books must be sent and returned by express, carefully packed, and the charges both ways must be paid by the borrower. The medical journals of which the library has duplicates may be sent and returned by mail. The Index Medicus is supplied to all posts in order that medical officers may be informed and make use of the latest additions to the library. Library S.G.O.

MEDICINES.

ARTICLES.	100	200	400	600	800	1,000
Acacia (pulvis), in 500-gm. bottles __botts.	2	3	4	5	6	6
Acetanilidum, 200-mgm. tablets (200 in bottle) __botts.	2	2	4	4	6	6
Acidum aceticum, in 250-c. c. bottles __botts.	1	1	1	2	2	2
Acidum arsenosum, 1-mgm. tablets (125 in bott.), for field use only_botts.	1	1	2	2	3	3
Acidum boricum (pulvis), in 250-gm. bottles __botts.	1	1	2	2	3	3
Acidum boricum, 324-mgm. tablets (125 in bott.), for field use only_botts.	1	1	2	2	3	3
Acidum carbolicum, in 250-gm. bottles __botts.	1	1	2	2	3	3
Acidum citricum, in 250-gm. bottles __botts.	1	1	2	2	3	3
Acidum gallicum, in 25-gm. bottles __botts.	1	1	1	2	2	2
Acidum hydrochloricum, in 250-c. c. g. s. bottles __botts.	1	1	2	2	3	3
Acidum hydrocyanicum dilutum, in 25-c. c. g. s. bottles __botts.	1	1	1	2	2	2
Acidum lacticum, in 25-c. c. g. s. bottles __botts.	1	1	1	2	2	2
Acidum nitricum, in 250-c. c. g. s. bottles __botts.	1	1	2	2	3	3
Acidum phosphoricum dilutum, in 250-c. c. g. s. bottles __botts.	1	1	1	2	2	2
Acidum salicylicum, in 250-gm. bottles __botts.	1	1	2	2	4	4
Acidum sulphuricum, in 250-c. c. g. s. bottles __botts.	1	1	2	2	3	3
Acidum sulphuricum aromaticum, in 250-c. c. g. s. bottles __botts.	1	1	2	2	3	3
Acidum tannicum, in 25-gm. bottles __botts.	2	2	3	3	4	4
Acidum tartaricum, in 250-gm. bottles __botts.	2	2	4	4	6	6
Aconiti tinctura, in 50-c. c. bottles __botts.	2	2	3	3	4	4
Aconiti tinctura, 0.1-c. c. tablets (200 in bottle) __botts.	1	1	1	2	2	2
Æther, in 500-c. c. tins __tins.	4	6	8	10	12	14
Ætheris spiritus compositus, in 250-c. c. bottles __botts.	1	1	2	2	3	3
Ætheris spiritus nitrosi, in 500-c. c. bottles __botts.	2	3	4	6	8	10
Alcohol, in 1-liter bottles __botts.	6	10	16	24	30	36
Aloe (pulvis), in 25-gm. bottles __botts.	2	2	3	3	4	4
Aloini pilulæ comp. (200 in bottle) __botts.	1	1	2	2	3	3
Alumen, in 250-gm. bottles __botts.	2	3	4	5	6	6
Alumen, 324-mgm. tablets (150 in bottle), for field use only __botts.	1	1	2	2	3	3
Ammoniæ aqua, 10 p. c., in 500-c. c. g. s. bottles __botts.	2	3	4	5	6	8
Ammoniæ spiritus aromaticus, in 250-c. c. bottles __botts.	1	2	3	4	5	6
Ammonii bromidum, in 250-gm. bottles __botts.	1	1	1	2	2	2
Ammonii carbonas, in 250-gm. bottles __botts.	1	1	2	2	3	3
Ammonii chloridi trochisci (100 in bottle) __botts.	2	3	4	6	8	10
Ammonii chloridum, in 250-gm. bottles __botts.	2	3	4	5	6	8
Amyl nitris (5-drop pearls), 12 in box __boxes.	2	2	3	3	4	4
Antimonii et potassii tartras, in 25-gm. bottles __botts.	1	1	1	1	1	1
Antipyrinum, 324-mgm. tablets (200 in bottle) __botts.	1	2	3	4	5	6
Apomorphinæ hydrochloras, 6-mgm. hypodermic tablets __tubes.	1	1	2	2	2	2
Argenti nitras, in crystals, in 25-gm. bottles __botts.	1	1	2	2	3	3
Argenti nitras fusus, in 25-gm. bottles __botts.	1	1	1	2	2	2
Asafœtida, in 25-gm. bottles __botts.	1	1	1	1	1	1
Aspidii oleoresina, in 50-c. c. bottles __botts.	1	1	1	1	1	1
Atropinæ sulphas, 0.65-mgm. hypodermic tablets __tubes.	1	1	2	2	2	2
Atropinæ sulphas, 0.13-mgm. ophthalmic discs. (50 in box) __boxes.	1	1	2	2	2	2
Belladonnæ emplastrum, in 2-meter tins __tins.	1	1	2	2	3	3
Belladonnæ foliorum extractum alcoholicum, in 25-gm. bottles__botts.	1	1	2	2	3	3
Bismuthi subnitras, in 500-gm. bottles __botts.	1	1	2	2	3	3
Buchu extractum fluidum, in 500-c. c. bottles __botts.	1	1	2	2	2	3
Caffeina, 65-mgm. hypodermic tablets __tubes.	1	1	2	2	2	2
Camphora, in 500-gm. bottles __botts.	1	1	2	2	3	3
Cannabis indicæ tinctura, 0.06-c. c. tablets (100 in bottle) __botts.	1	1	1	2	2	2

16

MEDICINES—Continued.

	ALLOWANCE FOR POSTS HAVING OFFICIAL POPULATION OF—					
	100	200	400	600	800	1,000
Cantharidis emplastrum, in 1-meter tins _____tins.	1	1	1	2	2	2
Cantharidis tinctura, in 100-c. c. bottles_____botts.	1	1	1	2	2	2
Capsici tinctura, in 100-c. c. bottles_____botts.	1	1	1	2	2	2
Capsicum, 32-mgm. tablets (150 in bottle), for field use only_____botts.	1	1	2	2	3	3
Cera flava, in 250-gm. cakes_____cakes.	1	1	1	2	2	2
Ceratum resinæ, in 250-gm. jars _____jars.	1	1	1	2	2	2
Cerii oxalas, in 25-gm. bottles_____botts.	1	1	1	2	2	2
Chloral, in 50-gm. g. s. bottles _____botts.	2	2	3	3	4	4
Chloroformum, in 250-c. c. bottles _____botts.	6	6	12	12	18	18
Chrysarobinum, in 25-gm. bottles_____botts.	1	1	1	1	1	1
Cinchonæ tinctura composita, in 500-c. c. bottles _____botts.	4	6	8	10	12	12
Cocainæ hydrochloras, in 5-gm. bottles _____botts.	1	1	2	2	3	3
Cocainæ hydrochloras, 10-mgm. hypodermic tablets _____tubes.	1	1	2	2	3	3
Colchici seminis extractum fluidum, in 50-c. c. bottles_____botts.	2	2	3	3	4	4
Collodium, in 50-c. c. bottles_____botts.	1	1	2	2	4	4
Coniinæ bromohydras, 0.65-mgm. hypodermic tablets _____tubes.	1	1	2	2	3	3
Copaiba, in 500-gm. bottles_____botts.	2	3	4	5	5	6
Copaibæ pilulæ comp. or tablets (100 in bottle)_____botts.	4	6	8	10	12	14
Creosotum, in 50-gm. g. s. bottles_____botts.	2	2	4	4	6	6
Creta præparata, in 250-gm. bottles_____botts.	1	1	2	2	3	3
Cupri arsenis, 0.325-mgm. tablets (200 in bottle) _____botts.	1	1	1	2	2	2
Cupri sulphas, in 50-gm. bottles_____botts.	1	1	1	1	1	1
Digitalinum, 1-mgm. hypodermic tablets _____tubes.	1	1	2	2	3	3
Digitalis tinctura, in 125-c. c. bottles_____botts.	2	2	3	3	4	4
Digitalis tinctura, 0.3-c. c. tablets (200 in bottle) _____botts.	2	3	4	6	6	8
Emplastrum (porous), in boxes of 24 _____boxes.	1	1	2	2	3	3
Ergotæ extractum fluidum, in 250-c. c. bottles_____botts.	1	2	3	4	5	6
Ergotinum, 130-mgm. tablets (200 in bottle)_____botts.	2	2	3	3	4	4
Eucalyptol, in 50-c. c. bottles_____botts.	2	2	3	3	4	4
Ferri chloridi tinctura, in 500-c. c. g. s. bottles_____botts.	1	2	3	4	5	6
Ferri et potassii tartras, in 250-gm. bottles_____botts.	1	1	2	2	2	2
Ferri et quininæ citras solubilis, in 100-gm. bottles_____botts.	1	2	3	4	5	6
Ferri iodidi syrupus, in 250-c. c. bottles_____botts.	1	1	2	2	3	3
Ferri pilulæ compositæ (200 in bottle)_____botts.	1	2	3	4	5	6
Ferri pyrophosphas solubilis, in 100-gm. bottles_____botts.	1	1	1	2	2	2
Ferri sulphas exsiccatus, in 100-gm. bottles_____botts.	1	1	1	2	2	2
Ferrum reductum, in 25-gm. bottles_____botts.	1	1	1	2	2	2
Gentianæ tinctura composita, in 500-c. c. bottles _____botts.	2	3	4	5	6	7
Glycerinum, in 500-c. c. bottles_____botts.	4	6	8	10	12	14
Glycyrrhizæ extractum purum (pulvis), in 250-gm. bottles _____botts.	2	3	4	6	8	10
Glycyrrhizæ mistura composita, tablets (400 in bottle) _____botts.	2	3	4	5	6	7
Glycyrrhizæ pulvis compositus, in 250-gm. bottles_____botts.	1	1	2	2	3	3
Hamamelidis extractum fluidum, in 250-c. c. bottles _____botts.	2	2	3	3	4	4
Hydrargyri chloridum corrosivum, in 100-gm. bottles_____botts.	1	1	1	1	1	1
Hydrargyri chloridum mite, in 100-gm. bottles_____botts.	1	1	2	2	3	3
Hydrargyri chloridum mite cum sodio bicarb., tablets (200 in bottle) _____botts.	2	3	4	5	6	8
Hydrargyri iodidum flavum, 10-mgm. tablets (200 in bottle)___botts.	2	3	4	5	6	8
Hydrargyri massa, in 100-gm. jars _____jars.	1	1	2	2	3	3
Hydrargyri massa, 324-mgm. tablets (125 in bott.) for field use only_botts.	1	1	2	2	3	3
Hydrargyri nitratis unguentum, in 100-gm. jars_____jars.	1	1	1	1	1	1
Hydrargyri oleatum, 10 per cent, in 500-gm. w. m. bottles _____botts.	1	1	1	2	2	2

MEDICINES—Continued.

ARTICLES.	100	200	400	600	800	1,000
Hydrargyri oxidum flavum, in 25-gm. bottles........................botts.	1	1	1	1	1	1
Hydrargyri unguentum, in 500-gm. jars..........................jars.	1	1	1	2	2	2
Hydrargyrum cum creta, in 100-gm. bottles......................botts.	1	1	2	2	3	3
Hydrastis extractum fluidum, in 250-c. c. bottles................botts.	1	1	1	2	2	2
Hydrogenii dioxidi aqua*..boxes.	1	1	1	2	2	2
Hyoscinæ hydrobromas, 0.65-mgm. hypodermic tablets.........tubes.	1	1	1	1	1	1
Hyoscyami extractum alcoholicum, in 25-gm. w. m. bottles....botts.	1	1	1	2	2	2
Hyoscyami pilulae compositæ (200 in bottle)....................botts.	1	1	2	2	3	3
Ichthyolum, in 25-gm. bottles....................................botts.	1	2	3	3	4	4
Iodoformum, in 100-gm. bottles..................................botts.	2	3	4	6	8	10
Iodum, in 50-gm. g. s. bottles...................................botts.	1	2	3	4	5	6
Ipecacuanha, 65-mgm. tablets (200 in bottle), for field use only..botts.	1	1	1	2	2	2
Ipecacuanha (pulvis), in 100-gm. bottles........................botts.	1	1	1	2	2	2
Ipecacuanhæ et opii pulvis, in 250-gm. bottles..................botts.	1	1	1	2	2	2
Ipecacuanhæ et opii pulvis, 324-mgm. tablets (200 in bottle)....botts.	1	1	2	2	3	3
Ipecacuanhæ extractum fluidum, in 250-c. c. bottles.......... botts.	1	1	2	2	3	3
Linimentum rubefaciens, tablets (50 in bottle), for field use only..botts.	2	2	3	3	4	4
Linum, in 2-kilo. tins..tins.	1	1	1	2	2	2
Linum (pulvis), in 4-kilo. tins..................................tins.	4	6	8	10	12	14
Lithii carbonas, in 25-gm. bottles..............................botts.	1	1	1	2	2	2
Lycopodium, in 50-gm. bottles..................................botts.	1	2	3	4	5	6
Magnesii carbonas, in 100-gm. papers.........................papers.	4	6	8	10	12	12
Magnesii sulphas, in 4-kilo. tins...............................tins.	1	2	3	4	5	6
Menthol, in 50-gm. bottles......................................botts.	1	1	2	2	3	3
Morphinæ sulphas, in 10-gm. bottles..........................botts.	2	4	6	8	10	12
Morphinæ sulphas, 8-mgm. hypodermic tablets.................tubes.	5	10	15	20	25	30
Morphinæ sulphas, 8-mgm. tablets (100 in bottle).............botts.	2	4	6	8	10	12
Myrrhæ tinctura, in 250-c. c. bottles...........................botts.	1	1	1	2	2	2
Nitroglycerinum, 0.65-mgm. hypodermic tablets...............tubes.	1	1	2	2	3	3
Nucis vomicæ extractum, in 25-gm. bottles....................botts.	1	1	2	2	3	3
Oleum caryophylli, in 25-c. c. bottles...........................botts.	1	1	1	1	1	1
Oleum gaultheriæ, in 100-c. c. bottles..........................botts.	1	1	2	2	3	3
Oleum gossypii seminis, in 1-liter bottles.......................botts.	12	24	36	48	60	72
Oleum menthæ piperitæ, in 100-c. c. bottles....................botts.	1	1	2	2	3	3
Oleum morrhuæ, in 500-c. c. bottles............................botts.	6	8	10	12	14	16
Oleum ricini, in 1-liter bottles..................................botts.	5	10	15	20	25	30
Oleum santali, in 100-c. c. bottles..............................botts.	1	1	2	2	3	3
Oleum terebinthinæ, in 1-liter bottles..........................botts.	2	4	6	8	10	12
Oleum theobromatis, in 250-gm. tins...........................tins.	1	1	2	2	3	3
Oleum tiglii, in 25-c. c. bottles.................................botts.	1	1	1	1	1	1
Oleum tiglii, 0.006-c. c. tablets (100 in bottle), for field use only..botts.	1	1	1	2	2	2
Opii pilulæ (or tablets), 65-mgm. (200 in bottle)...............botts.	1	2	3	4	5	6
Opii tinctura, in 500-c. c. bottles...............................botts.	1	2	3	4	5	6
Opii tinctura camphorata, in 500-c. c. bottles...................botts.	4	8	12	16	20	24
Opii tinctura camphorata, 0.4-c. c. tablets (200 in bottle).......botts.	1	2	3	4	5	6
Opium (pulvis), in 100-gm. bottles..............................botts.	1	1	1	2	2	2
Pepsinum, in 50-gm. bottles....................................botts.	2	3	4	6	8	10
Petrolatum liquidum, in 500-gm. bottles........................botts.	1	2	3	4	5	6
Petrolatum spissum, 48.8 C., in 500-gm. tins...................tins.	4	6	8	12	16	20
Phenacetinum, 324-mgm. tablets (200 in bottle)................botts.	1	2	3	4	5	6

*Each box contains all materials necessary to make three liters of a three per cent or ten volumes solution.

18

MEDICINES—Continued.

ARTICLES.	ALLOWANCE FOR POSTS HAVING OFFICIAL POPULATION OF—					
	100	200	400	600	800	1,000
Physostigmatis tinctura, 0.06-c. c. tablets (100 in bottle) _____ botts.	1	1	1	1	1	1
Physostigminæ sulphas, 1-mgm. hypodermic tablets _____ tubes.	1	1	1	1	1	1
Physostigminæ sulphas, 0.0325-mgm. ophthalmic discs (50 in box)_box.	1	1	1	1	2	2
Pilocarpi extractum fluidum, in 250-c. c. bottles _____ botts.	1	1	2	2	3	3
Pilulæ camphoræ et opii (or tablets), (200 in bottle) _____ botts.	2	3	4	5	6	7
Pilulæ carminativæ (200 in bottle) _____ botts.	2	3	4	5	6	7
Pilulæ catharticæ compositæ (or tablets), (200 in bottle) _____ botts.	3	4	6	8	10	12
Plumbi acetas, in 500-gm. bottles _____ botts.	1	1	2	2	3	3
Plumbi acetas, 130-mgm. tablets (100 in bottle), for field use only _botts.	1	1	1	2	2	2
Podophylli resina, in 25-gm. bottles _____ botts.	1	1	1	2	2	2
Podophylli resina, 16-mgm. tablets (100 in bottle), for field use only _____ botts.	1	1	1	2	2	2
Potassa, in 25-gm. bottles _____ botts.	2	2	2	4	4	4
Potassii acetas, in 500-gm. bottles _____ botts.	1	1	2	2	3	3
Potassii arsenitis liquor, in 250-c. c. bottles _____ botts.	1	1	2	2	3	3
Potassii bicarbonas, in 500-gm. bottles _____ botts.	1	1	2	2	3	3
Potassii bromidum, in 500-gm. bottles _____ botts.	1	2	3	4	5	6
Potassii chloras, in 500-gm. bottles _____ botts.	2	3	4	5	6	7
Potassii chloras, 324-mgm. tablets (200 in bottle), for field use only_botts.	2	3	4	5	6	7
Potassii et sodii tartras (pulvis), in 500-gm. bottles _____ botts.	4	6	8	10	12	14
Potassii iodidum, in 500-gm. bottles _____ botts.	1	2	3	4	5	6
Potassii iodidum, 324-mgm. tablets (200 in bottle), for field use only _____ botts.	1	1	1	2	2	2
Potassii permanganas, in 50-gm. bottles _____ botts.	1	1	2	2	3	3
Pruni virgiuianæ extractum fluidum, in 500-c. c. bottles _____ botts.	1	1	1	2	2	2
Quininæ hydrochloras, 32-mgm. hypodermic tablets _____ tubes.	2	2	3	3	4	4
Quininæ sulphas, in 25-gm. bottles _____ botts.	12	18	24	32	48	60
Quininæ sulphas, 200-mgm. tablets (500 in bottle) _____ botts.	4	6	8	10	12	14
Rhamni purshianæ extractum fluidum, in 500-c. c. bottles _____ botts.	1	1	2	2	3	3
Rhei extractum fluidum, in 250-c. c. bottles _____ botts.	1	1	1	2	2	2
Rheum (pulvis), in 50-gm. bottles _____ botts.	1	1	2	2	3	3
Saccharum lactis (pulvis), in 100-gm. bottles _____ botts.	1	1	2	2	3	3
Salol, 324-mgm. tablets (125 in bottle) _____ botts.	2	2	3	3	4	4
Salophen, in 50-gm. bottles _____ botts.	1	1	2	2	3	3
Santoninum, 32-mgm. tablets (50 in bottle) _____ botts.	1	1	1	2	2	2
Scillæ syrupus, in 500-c. c. bottles _____ botts.	4	8	12	16	20	24
Sinapis emplastrum, in 4-meter tins _____ tins.	1	1	2	2	3	3
Sinapis nigra (pulvis), in 500-gm. tins _____ tins.	4	6	8	10	12	14
Sodii bicarbonas, in 500-gm. bottles _____ botts.	4	6	8	10	12	14
Sodii bicarbonas, 324-mgm. tablets (200 in bottle), for field use only _____ botts.	1	1	1	2	2	2
Sodii bicarb. et menthæ pip. (tablets), 250 in bottle _____ botts.	1	2	3	4	5	6
Sodii boras (pulvis), in 500-gm. bottles _____ botts.	1	2	3	3	4	4
Sodii bromidum, in 250-gm. bottles _____ botts.	1	1	2	2	3	3
Sodii hyposulphis, in 250-gm. bottles _____ botts.	1	1	2	2	3	3
Sodii phosphas, in 100-gm. bottles _____ botts.	1	1	2	2	3	3
Sodii salicylas, in 500-gm. bottles _____ botts.	2	3	4	5	6	7
Sodii salicylas, 324-mgm. tablets (200 in bottle) _____ botts.	2	3	4	5	6	8
Strophanthi tinctura, in 100-c. c. bottles _____ botts.	1	1	1	2	2	2
Strychninæ sulphas, 1-mgm. tablets (500 in bottle) _____ botts.	2	2	3	3	4	4

MEDICINES—Continued.

ARTICLES.

ARTICLES.		ALLOWANCE FOR POSTS HAVING OFFICIAL POPULATION OF—					
		100	200	400	600	800	1,000
Sulphonal, 324-mgm. tablets (200 in bottle) _____botts.		2	2	4	4	6	6
Sulphur lotum, in 250-gm. bottles_____botts.		1	1	1	2	2	2
Terebenum, in 250-c. c. bottles_____botts.		1	1	2	2	3	3
Thymol, in 25-gm. bottles _____botts.		1	1	1	2	2	2
Tolutanum balsamum, in 250-gm. bottles_____botts.		1	1	2	2	3	3
Valerianæ extractum fluidum, in 250-c. c. bottles_____botts.		1	1	1	2	2	2
Veratri viridis tinctura, in 100-c. c. bottles _____botts.		1	1	1	1	1	1
Zinci oxidum, in 250-gm. bottles_____botts.		1	1	1	2	2	2
Zinci sulphas, in 500-gm. bottles_____botts.		1	1	1	2	2	2
Zinci sulphas, 324-mgm. tablets (100 in bottle), for field use only_botts.		1	1	1	2	2	2
Zingiberis extractum fluidum, in 250 c. c. bottles _____botts.		2	2	3	4	5	6

ANTISEPTICS AND DISINFECTANTS.

ARTICLES.		ALLOWANCE FOR POSTS HAVING OFFICIAL POPULATION OF—					
		100	200	400	600	800	1,000
Acid, carbolic, crude (U. S. P.), in 1-kilo. bottles _____botts.		10	15	20	25	30	35
Antiseptic tablets (200 in bottle)_____botts.		2	2	3	3	4	4
Iron sulphate, commercial, in 10-kilo. boxes _____boxes.		5	10	20	30	40	50
Lime, chloride, in 500-gm. w. m. bottles _____botts.		10	15	20	25	30	35
Mercury, corrosive chloride, in 500-gm. bottles _____botts..		1	2	3	4	5	6
Soda, chlorinated solution (6 per cent available chlorine), in 500 c. c. bottles_____botts.		1	1	1	2	2	2
Sulphur, in roll _____kilos.		10	15	20	25	30	35
Tricresol *, in 1-kilo. bottles_____botts.		2	3	5	6	7	8

* Tricresol will be issued in lieu of crude carbolic acid if desired.

HOSPITAL STORES.

ARTICLES.		ALLOWANCE FOR POSTS HAVING OFFICIAL POPULATION OF—					
		100	200	400	600	800	1,000
Beef extract, in 100-gm. tins or jars_____tins.		10	15	20	25	30	35
Brandy, in 1-liter bottles_____botts.		2	4	6	8	10	12
Soap, Castile or its equivalent _____kilos.		2	3	4	5	6	7
Soap, common_____kilos.		5	8	10	12	14	16
Sugar, white, in 6-kilo. tins_____tins.		1	2	3	4	5	6
Whisky, in 1-liter bottles _____botts.		6	8	12	16	20	24

MICROSCOPICAL ACCESSORIES.

ARTICLES.		Allowance for Posts having Official Population of—					
		100	200	400	600	800	1,000
Agar-agar	kilos.			1	1	1	1
Aniline oil, in 125-c. c. bottles	botts.	1	1	1	2	2	2
Balsam bottle	no.	1	1	1	1	1	1
Bismarck brown, in 4-gm. bottles	botts.	1	1	1	1	1	1
Canada balsam, in 30-c. c. bottles	botts.	1	1	1	2	2	2
Carmine, in 15-gm. bottles	botts.	1	1	1	1	1	1
Eosin, in 15-gm. bottles	botts.	1	1	1	1	1	1
Fuchsin, in 15-gm. bottles	botts.	1	1	1	1	1	1
Gelatin	kilos.			1	1	1	1
Gentian violet, in 15-gm. bottles	botts.	1	1	1	1	1	1
Glass covers, 16 or 19 mm. square	gms.	30	30	30	30	30	30
Glass slides, 25 x 75 mm	doz.	4	4	4	8	8	8
Hæmatoxylon, in 8-gm. bottles	botts.	1	1	1	1	1	1
Methyl blue, in 15-gm. bottles	botts.	1	1	1	1	1	1
Oil of cedar, in 30-c. c. bottles	botts.	1	1	1	1	1	1
Peptone	kilos.			¼	¼	¼	¼
Paraffin, in ¼-kilo. cakes	cakes.	1	1	1	1	1	1
Xylenum, in 250-c. c. bottles	botts.	1	1	1	2	2	2

STATIONERY.

ARTICLES.		Allowance for Posts having Official Population of—					
		100	200	400	600	800	1,000
Blank books, cap, 4-quire	no.	4	4	4	6	6	6
Blank books, 8mo., 4-quire	no.	2	2	3	3	4	4
Blotters, hand	no.	2	2	2	2	2	2
Elastic bands, assorted	gross.	2	2	2	3	3	4
Envelopes, official, large	no.	100	100	100	150	150	150
Envelopes, official, letter	no.	400	400	500	500	600	600
Envelopes, official, note	no.	100	100	100	150	200	200
Erasers, steel	no.	2	2	2	2	2	2
India rubber	pieces.	2	2	3	3	4	4
Ink, writing, in 1-liter bottles	botts.	2	2	3	3	4	4
Ink, carmine, in 30-c. c. bottles	botts.	2	2	3	3	4	4
Mucilage	botts.	2	3	4	5	6	7
Pads, prescription	no.	18	24	36	36	48	48
Pads, letter	no.	6	8	10	12	14	16
Paper, blotting	qrs.	1	1	1	2	2	2
Paper fasteners	boxes.	1	1	1	1	1	1
Paper, writing, legal cap	qrs.	6	6	8	8	10	10
Paper, writing, letter	qrs.	16	16	18	18	24	24
Paper, writing, letter, typewriter	qrs.			18	20	24	24
Paper, writing, note	qrs.	6	6	6	12	12	12
Pencils, lead	no.	18	18	24	24	36	36
Penholders	no.	8	8	10	10	12	12
Pens, steel. (See par. 36.)	no.	96	96	144	144	192	192
Ribbons, copying, for typewriter, as required. (See par. 43.)	no.						
Ribbons, record, for typewriter, as required. (See par. 43.)	no.						

21

SURGICAL INSTRUMENTS, APPLIANCES, AND DRESSINGS.

ARTICLES.		ALLOWANCE FOR POSTS HAVING OFFICIAL POPULATION OF—					
		100	200	400	600	800	1,000
Apparatus, compressed air	no.	1	1	1	1	1	1
Apparatus, electric*	no.	1	1	1	1	1	1
Apparatus, restraint	no.	1	1	1	1	1	1
Apparatus, steam sterilizing	no.	1	1	1	1	1	1
Atomizers, hand	no.	2	2	3	3	4	4
Bags, rubber, hot-water	no.	1	1	1	2	2	2
Bags, rubber, ice, spinal	no.	1	1	1	2	2	2
Bandages, roller, assorted, in boxes of 8 dozen	boxes.	3	4	5	7	9	12
Bandages, rubber (Martin's), 4 meters by 63 mm	no.	1	1	1	2	2	2
Bandages, suspensory	no.	4	6	8	10	12	16
Bougies, flexible, as required	no.						
Boxes, fracture, folding	no.	1	1	1	2	2	2
Brush holders for larynx	no.	1	1	1	2	2	2
Case, aspirating	no.	1	1	1	1	1	1
Case, capital operating	no.	1	1	1	1	1	1
Case, dental †	no.	1	1	1	1	1	1
Case, emergency. (See par. 46.)	no.						
Case, eye and ear	no.	1	1	1	1	1	1
Case, field. (See par. 46.)	no.						
Case, field operating, when specially approved	no.	1	1	1	1	1	1
Case, forceps, hæmostatic, 12 in set	no.	1	1	1	1	1	1
Case, genito-urethral	no.	1	1	1	1	1	1
Case, genito-urinary	no.	1	1	1	1	1	1
Case, minor operating	no.	1	1	1	1	1	1
Case, obstetrical and gynecological	no.	1	1	1	1	1	1
Case, pocket, personal or post	no.	1	1	2	2	2	3
Case, pocket, aseptic ‡	no.	1	1	2	2	2	3
Case, post-mortem	no.	1	1	1	1	1	1
Case, stomach pump	no.	1	1	1	1	1	1
Case, tooth extracting	no.	1	1	1	1	1	1
Case, trial lenses	no.			1	1	1	1
Catheter box	no.	1	1	1	1	1	1
Catheters, flexible, as required	no.						
Cotton, absorbent	kilos.	1	2	3	3	4	4
Cotton, styptic, in 30-gm. packages	pkgs.	1	1	1	1	2	2
Cotton bats	kilos.	2	3	4	6	8	9
Curettes, as required	no.						
First-aid packets. (See pars. 35 and 41.)	no.	12	18	24	36	48	60
Forceps, needle (Tiemann's)	no.	1	1	1	1	1	1
Gauze, plain	meters.	20	30	40	60	80	100
Inflator, Politzer's	no.	1	1	1	1	1	1
Inhaler and vaporizer	no.	1	1	1	1	1	1
Inhaler, ether	no.	1	1	1	1	1	1
Lavage tubes	no.	1	1	1	1	2	2
Ligatures, catgut, sterilized, in alcohol, 3 sizes, 1 meter each, in bottles	botts.	2	2	3	3	4	5
Ligature silk	gms.	15	15	30	30	45	45
Microscope	no.	1	1	1	1	1	1

*Sulphuric acid, sulphate of copper, and bichromate of potash in 500-gramme bottles, and metallic mercury in 125-gramme bottles, will be issued as required for battery use.
† Will not be issued to posts near which the services of a dentist may be obtained.
‡ This pattern of pocket case will not be issued for post use until the supply of personal and post cases is exhausted.

22

SURGICAL INSTRUMENTS, APPLIANCES, AND DRESSINGS—Continued.

ARTICLES.

<table>
<tr><th rowspan="2">ARTICLES.</th><th colspan="6">ALLOWANCE FOR POSTS HAVING OFFICIAL POPULATION OF—</th></tr>
<tr><th>100</th><th>200</th><th>400</th><th>600</th><th>800</th><th>1,000</th></tr>
<tr><td>Microtome, large ____no.</td><td></td><td></td><td>1</td><td>1</td><td>1</td><td>1</td></tr>
<tr><td>Muslin, unbleached____meters.</td><td>5</td><td>5</td><td>10</td><td>10</td><td>15</td><td>15</td></tr>
<tr><td>Needles, common, assorted____papers.</td><td>1</td><td>1</td><td>1</td><td>2</td><td>2</td><td>2</td></tr>
<tr><td>Needles, surgical, assorted, as required ____no.</td><td></td><td></td><td></td><td></td><td></td><td></td></tr>
<tr><td>Needles, surgical (Hagedorn's), 20 in set____sets.</td><td>1</td><td>1</td><td>1</td><td>1</td><td>1</td><td>1</td></tr>
<tr><td>Oakum or its equivalent____kilos.</td><td>5</td><td>8</td><td>10</td><td>12</td><td>15</td><td>20</td></tr>
<tr><td>Paper, dressing, oiled, in 24-meter rolls ____rolls.</td><td>1</td><td>1</td><td>2</td><td>3</td><td>4</td><td>5</td></tr>
<tr><td>Pins, assorted____papers.</td><td>4</td><td>6</td><td>8</td><td>10</td><td>12</td><td>15</td></tr>
<tr><td>Pins, safety, 3 sizes____dozen.</td><td>3</td><td>3</td><td>6</td><td>6</td><td>8</td><td>10</td></tr>
<tr><td>Plaster, adhesive, 30 cm. wide, in 5-meter rolls ____meters.</td><td>20</td><td>25</td><td>30</td><td>40</td><td>50</td><td>60</td></tr>
<tr><td>Plaster, isinglass, in 1-meter rolls____meters.</td><td>2</td><td>2</td><td>4</td><td>4</td><td>6</td><td>6</td></tr>
<tr><td>Plaster of Paris, in 2-kilo. tins____kilos.</td><td>4</td><td>4</td><td>6</td><td>10</td><td>12</td><td>14</td></tr>
<tr><td>Pouches, Hospital Corps. (See par. 46.)____no.</td><td></td><td></td><td></td><td></td><td></td><td></td></tr>
<tr><td>Pouches, orderly ____no.</td><td>1</td><td>1</td><td>1</td><td>1</td><td>2</td><td>2</td></tr>
<tr><td>Probangs ____no.</td><td>4</td><td>4</td><td>6</td><td>6</td><td>10</td><td>10</td></tr>
<tr><td>Rubber sheeting____meters.</td><td>4</td><td>4</td><td>6</td><td>6</td><td>8</td><td>8</td></tr>
<tr><td>Scarificator ____no.</td><td>1</td><td>1</td><td>1</td><td>1</td><td>1</td><td>1</td></tr>
<tr><td>Silk, gray, for shades____meters.</td><td>¼</td><td>¼</td><td>½</td><td>½</td><td>1</td><td>1</td></tr>
<tr><td>Silk, oiled, in 5-meter rolls ____meters.</td><td>5</td><td>5</td><td>10</td><td>10</td><td>15</td><td>15</td></tr>
<tr><td>Speculum, rectal ____no.</td><td>1</td><td>1</td><td>1</td><td>1</td><td>1</td><td>1</td></tr>
<tr><td>Splints, felt for ____pieces.</td><td>4</td><td>6</td><td>8</td><td>8</td><td>10</td><td>10</td></tr>
<tr><td>Sponge holders for throat ____no.</td><td>1</td><td>1</td><td>1</td><td>2</td><td>2</td><td>2</td></tr>
<tr><td>Sponges, chloroform ____no.</td><td>1</td><td>1</td><td>1</td><td>2</td><td>2</td><td>2</td></tr>
<tr><td>Sponges, small, in strings of 50 ____no.</td><td>50</td><td>50</td><td>50</td><td>100</td><td>100</td><td>100</td></tr>
<tr><td>Sprinklers, iodoform, h. r____no.</td><td>1</td><td>1</td><td>1</td><td>2</td><td>2</td><td>2</td></tr>
<tr><td>Stethoscope ____no.</td><td>1</td><td>1</td><td>1</td><td>1</td><td>1</td><td>1</td></tr>
<tr><td>Stethoscope, double____no.</td><td>1</td><td>1</td><td>1</td><td>1</td><td>1</td><td>1</td></tr>
<tr><td>Surgical pump____no.</td><td></td><td></td><td>1</td><td>1</td><td>1</td><td>1</td></tr>
<tr><td>Syringes, hypodermic____no.</td><td>1</td><td>1</td><td>2</td><td>2</td><td>2</td><td>3</td></tr>
<tr><td>Syringes, rubber, self-injecting, bulb ____no.</td><td>1</td><td>4</td><td>4</td><td>6</td><td>6</td><td>6</td></tr>
<tr><td>Syringes, rubber, self-injecting, fountain____no.</td><td>2</td><td>2</td><td>2</td><td>3</td><td>3</td><td>3</td></tr>
<tr><td>Tape, cotton ____pieces.</td><td>2</td><td>2</td><td>3</td><td>3</td><td>4</td><td>5</td></tr>
<tr><td>Tents, laminaria or tupelo ____no.</td><td>6</td><td>6</td><td>12</td><td>12</td><td>18</td><td>18</td></tr>
<tr><td>Thermo-cautery (Paquelin's) *____no.</td><td></td><td></td><td>1</td><td>1</td><td>1</td><td>1</td></tr>
<tr><td>Thermometers, clinical. (See par. 42.)____no.</td><td>2</td><td>2</td><td>2</td><td>3</td><td>3</td><td>4</td></tr>
<tr><td>Thread, cotton, assorted ____spools.</td><td>2</td><td>2</td><td>3</td><td>3</td><td>4</td><td>4</td></tr>
<tr><td>Thread, linen, unbleached ____gms.</td><td>30</td><td>30</td><td>30</td><td>60</td><td>60</td><td>60</td></tr>
<tr><td>Tongue depressors____no.</td><td>1</td><td>1</td><td>1</td><td>2</td><td>2</td><td>2</td></tr>
<tr><td>Tourniquet and bandage, rubber ____no.</td><td>1</td><td>1</td><td>1</td><td>1</td><td>1</td><td>1</td></tr>
<tr><td>Tourniquets, field. (See par. 41.)____no.</td><td></td><td></td><td></td><td></td><td></td><td></td></tr>
<tr><td>Trusses, single____no.</td><td>2</td><td>3</td><td>4</td><td>6</td><td>6</td><td>8</td></tr>
<tr><td>Trusses, double ____no.</td><td>1</td><td>1</td><td>1</td><td>2</td><td>2</td><td>2</td></tr>
<tr><td>Tubes, drainage, Nos. 1, 2, and 3 of each ____meters.</td><td>1</td><td>1</td><td>1</td><td>1</td><td>1</td><td>1</td></tr>
<tr><td>Vision test set ____no.</td><td>1</td><td>1</td><td>1</td><td>1</td><td>1</td><td>1</td></tr>
<tr><td>Wire, suture, silver, in loops ____loops.</td><td>1</td><td>1</td><td>1</td><td>2</td><td>2</td><td>2</td></tr>
</table>

* Benzine, of a specific gravity not greater than 0.724, in 1-liter bottles, will be issued as required for use with this cautery.

FURNITURE, BEDDING, AND CLOTHING.

ARTICLES.	Allowance for Posts having Official Population of—					
	100	200	400	600	800	1,000
Basin, wash, delf, for office ....no.	1	1	1	1	1	1
Basins, wash hand, agate ware ....no.	6	6	6	10	10	10
Baskets, letter........no.	2	2	2	2	2	2
Baskets, waste-paper........no.	2	2	2	2	2	2
Bath tubs ....no.	2	2	2	2	3	3
Bed cradles ....no.	1	1	2	2	3	3
Beds, invalid........no.	1	1	1	1	2	2
Bedsteads, with woven-wire mattresses........no.	12	12	18	18	30	30
Bedstead casters, rubber, for beds in wards only, as required ....no.						
Bell, call ....no.	1	1	1	1	1	1
Blanket cases, for field use only* ....no.						
Blankets, gray, for field use only, as required ....no.						
Blankets, white ....no.	40	50	70	100	100	100
Bookcases........no.	1	1	1	2	2	2
Cabinet for blanks ....no.	1	1	1	1	1	1
Chairs, arm ....no.	10	12	15	20	25	30
Chairs, common........no.	10	12	15	20	25	30
Chairs, invalid, rolling ....no.	1	1	1	2	2	2
Chairs, office, revolving ....no.	1	1	1	2	2	2
Chairs, rocking........no.	3	3	4	5	6	6
Clocks†........no.	3	3	3	4	4	4
Close stools ....no.	1	1	2	2	3	4
Commodes, earth closet........no.	1	1	2	2	3	3
Cups, sponge ....no.	2	2	2	2	2	2
Cuspidors........no.	6	6	10	10	15	15
Desks, office ....no.	1	1	1	2	2	2
Desks, office, cloth or rubber duck top for, as required ....no.						
Dish, soap, with cover, for office ....no.	1	1	1	1	1	1
Holland, for curtains, as required ....meters.						
Inkstands ....no.	3	3	3	4	4	4
Lamps, hand ....no.	2	2	2	3	3	3
Lamps, stand........no.	2	2	2	3	3	3
Linoleum, as required........meters.						
Looking-glasses ....no.	4	4	6	6	8	8
Mats, door, manila........no.	4	4	6	6	8	8
Mats, door, woven wire ....no.	3	3	4	4	5	8
Matting, cocoa, as required. (See par. 50.)........meters.						
Matting, cocoa, zinc ends for, as required. (See par. 50.)........no.						
Mattress covers ....no.	6	6	10	10	16	15
Mattresses, hair, sectional. (See par. 31.)........no.	10	12	18	24	30	40
Mosquito bars, as required ....no.						
Oilcloth for table........meters.	6	6	6	12	12	12
Paper cutters ....no.	2	2	2	2	2	2
Paperweights ....no.	2	2	2	2	2	2
Penracks........no.	3	3	3	3	3	3
Pillows, feather........no.	6	6	6	12	12	12
Pillows, hair ....no.	15	24	30	40	50	60
Pillow cases, cotton........no.	40	40	60	80	100	130
Pitcher, delf, for office ....no.	1	1	1	1	1	1
Pitcher, ice, silver plated........no.	1	1	1	1	1	1

* Issued in the proportion of one case to ten gray blankets.
† Clocks will be issued on the basis of one for each ward, one for kitchen, and one for dispensary.

FURNITURE, BEDDING, AND CLOTHING—Continued.

ARTICLES.	ALLOWANCE FOR POSTS HAVING OFFICIAL POPULATION OF—					
	100	200	400	600	800	1,000
Quilts, colored _____no.	12	12	18	24	30	36
Quilts, white_____no.	12	12	18	24	30	36
Refrigerators_____no.	1	1	1	2	2	2
Rulers_____no.	2	2	2	2	2	2
Safe, iron_____no.	1	1	1	1	1	1
Screens, bed, folding, frames for. (See par. 48.)_____no.	2	2	2	4	4	4
Screens, door, wire, as required. (See par. 47.)_____no.						
Screens, window, wire, as required. (See par. 47.)_____no.						
Screens, wire netting for, as required. (See par. 47.)_____meters.						
Sheets, cotton_____no.	40	50	75	100	125	150
Shirts, cotton_____no.	20	20	40	40	50	60
Slippers_____pairs.	12	12	18	18	24	36
Splints, anterior (Smith's)_____no.	2	2	2	2	2	2
Stamp, penalty, rubber_____no.	1	1	1	1	1	1
Tablecloths, linen_____meters.	15	15	20	25	30	35
Tables, bedside_____no.	12	12	18	18	30	30
Tables, dining, extension_____no.	1	1	1	1	2	2
Towels, hand_____doz.	4	8	12	15	18	20
Towels, roller_____doz.	1	1	2	3	4	5
Typewriter_____no.			1	1	1	1
Water coolers_____no.	2	2	2	3	3	3
Window curtains, as required_____no.						
Window curtain fixtures, as required_____sets.						

MISCELLANEOUS.

ARTICLES.	ALLOWANCE FOR POSTS HAVING OFFICIAL POPULATION OF—					
	100	200	400	600	800	1,000
Bacteriological set, as per list. (See par. 52.)_____no.			1	1	1	1
Bandage winder_____no.	1	1	1	1	1	1
Bath bricks_____no.	2	2	4	4	6	6
Bedpans, delf or agate ware_____no.	2	3	4	5	5	6
Blowers for insect powder_____no.	1	1	1	1	2	2
Boiler, tin_____no.	1	1	1	1	1	1
Boilers, double, for cooking_____no.	1	1	1	1	2	2
Bowls, chopping_____no.	1	1	1	1	1	1
Bowls, soup, delf_____no.	18	24	36	48	60	72
Bowls, sugar, with lid_____no.	2	2	4	4	6	6
Boxes, ointment, impervious_____doz.	12	15	20	25	30	35
Boxes, pill_____doz.	20	25	30	40	50	60
Boxes, powder_____doz.	18	18	24	30	36	48
Brooms_____no.	12	18	24	36	48	48
Brooms, whisk_____no.	2	2	2	2	2	2
Brushes, dust_____no.	2	2	4	4	6	6
Brushes, flesh, rubber_____no.	1	1	1	1	2	2
Brushes, nail_____no.	1	1	1	1	2	2
Brushes, nail, holder for_____no.	1	1	1	1	1	1
Brushes, scrubbing_____no.	12	12	18	18	24	24

25

MISCELLANEOUS--Continued.

ARTICLES.	ALLOWANCE FOR POSTS HAVING OFFICIAL POPULATION OF—					
	100	200	400	600	800	1,000
Brushes, stove-blacking_____no.	3	3	3	4	4	4
Buckets, covered, 7-liter_____no.	2	2	4	4	5	6
Buckets, fiber_____no.	4	6	8	10	12	15
Buckets, fire, galvanized iron _____no.	12	12	18	18	24	24
Burner, Bunsen's *_____no.	1	1	1	1	1	1
Can openers_____no.	2	2	2	2	2	2
Candlesticks _____no.	2	2	2	2	2	2
Cans, milk, 9-liter_____no.	1	1	2	2	2	3
Capsules, gelatin, 100 in box, 4 sizes_____boxes.	10	12	16	20	24	30
Casters_____no.	1	1	2	2	2	2
Chamois skins _____no.	2	2	3	3	4	4
Charts, anatomical, in case_____set.	1	1	1	1	1	1
Chemical set, as per list. (See par. 52.) _____no.			1	1	1	1
Cleaver_____no.	1	1	1	1	1	1
Clothes baskets_____no.	2	2	2	3	4	4
Clothes line, manila_____meters.	60	60	60	90	90	90
Colanders_____no.	1	1	1	2	2	2
Cork borers, set of 6 _____set.	1	1	1	1	1	1
Cork extractor_____no.	1	1	1	1	1	1
Cork presser _____no.	1	1	1	1	1	1
Corks, assorted, in bags of 24 dozen _____doz.	48	48	96	96	144	144
Corks, large (No. 10) _____doz.	2	2	3	3	4	4
Corkscrews_____no.	2	2	2	3	3	3
Crutches _____pairs.	4	4	6	6	8	8
Crutches, rubber tips for _____no.	8	8	12	12	16	16
Cups _____no.	18	24	36	48	60	72
Cups, feeding _____no.	2	4	6	8	10	12
Cups, spit_____no.	4	6	8	10	12	15
Cushions, rubber, small_____no.	2	2	2	3	3	3
Cushions, rubber, with open center_____no.	1	1	1	2	2	2
Cutting pliers, for fixed bandages _____no.	1	1	1	1	1	1
Dippers _____no.	3	3	4	4	5	5
Dish covers, wire netting, assorted_____no.	6	6	9	9	12	12
Dishes, meat, assorted _____no.	6	6	8	8	12	12
Dishes, vegetable, with covers _____no.	4	4	6	8	10	12
Dispensing set. (See page 29.) _____set.	1	1	1	1	1	1
Dispensing set, labels for _____set.	1	1	1	1	1	1
Drawer pulls, with labels, as required _____no.						
Dusters, feather, long handle _____no.	1	1	1	2	2	2
Dusters, feather, short handle _____no.	2	2	3	3	4	4
Egg beater _____no.	1	1	1	1	1	1
Envelopes for tablets, 5 x 6 cm _____doz.	20	25	30	35	40	50
Eye shades_____no.	2	2	3	3	4	4
Fans _____no.	12	12	18	18	24	24
Fire extinguishers (force pump)_____no.	1	1	1	2	2	2
Flasks, 500-c. c._____no.	2	2	3	3	4	4
Flasks, 1,000-c. c_____no.	2	2	3	3	4	4
Forks, carving _____no.	2	2	2	3	3	3
Forks, flesh _____no.	1	1	1	2	2	2
Forks, table, common. (See par. 51.)_____no.						
Forks, table, silver plated. (See par. 51.)_____no.	24	36	48	56	72	72

* Will not be issued to posts that have no gas supply.

MISCELLANEOUS—Continued.

ARTICLES.	\multicolumn{6}{c}{ALLOWANCE FOR POSTS HAVING OFFICIAL POPULATION OF—}
	100	200	400	600	800	1,000
Funnels, glass, ¼, ½, and 1 liter, of each_____no.	1	1	1	2	2	2
Glue, liquid, in ¼-liter cans_____cans.	1	1	1	2	2	2
Grater, large_____no.	1	1	1	1	1	1
Graters, small._____no.	1	1	1	2	2	2
Gravy boats_____no.	2	2	4	4	5	6
Gridirons_____no.	1	1	2	2	2	2
Grindstone, complete, 25-cm., kitchen_____no.	1	1	1	1	1	1
Hammer_____no.	1	1				
Hand grenades_____no.	12	18	24	36	48	48
Hatchets_____no.	1	1				
Hone_____no.	1	1	1	1	1	1
Hose, canvas, 2.5-cm., in 15-meter lengths_____meters.	30	30	30	60	60	60
Hose nozzles, plain and spray, of each_____no.	1	1	1	1	1	1
Hose, reel cart for_____no.	1	1	1	1	1	1
Insect powder, in ½-kilo. tins_____kilos.	1	1	2	2	3	3
Kettles, tea_____no.	2	2	2	3	3	3
Knives, bread_____no.	1	1	1	2	2	2
Knives, butcher's_____no.	1	1	1	2	2	2
Knives, carving_____no.	2	2	2	3	3	3
Knives, chopping_____no.	1	1	1	1	1	1
Knives, table, common. (See par. 51.)_____no.						
Knives, table, silver plated. (See par. 51.)_____no.	24	36	48	56	72	72
Labels for vials_____gross.	2	3	4	5	6	7
Ladder, step_____no.	1	1	1	1	1	1
Ladles_____no.	2	2	2	3	3	3
Lamp chimneys, as required *_____no.						
Lamp shades, as required_____no.						
Lamps, spirit, glass_____no.	1	1	1	2	2	2
Lamp wicks, as required *_____no.						
Lantern glasses, extra, red or white, as required_____no.						
Lantern wicks, as required_____no.						
Lanterns_____no.	2	2	2	3	3	3
Lawn mower_____no.	1	1	1	1	1	1
Litters_____no.	2	2	3	3	4	5
Litters, canvas for, as required. (See par. 39.)_____pieces.						
Litters, straps for, as required_____no.						
Litter slings, as required_____pairs.						
Lye, concentrated, in ½-kilo. tins_____kilos.	3	4	5	6	7	8
Measures, ¼ to ½ liter_____set.	1	1	1	1	1	1
Measures, graduated, glass, 500-c. c_____no.	2	2	2	2	2	3
Measures, graduated, glass, 250-c. c_____no.	2	2	2	3	3	3
Measures, graduated, glass, 100-c. c_____no.	2	2	2	3	3	3
Meat cutter_____no.	1	1	1	1	1	1
Medicine droppers_____no.	12	12	24	24	36	48
Medicine glasses_____no.	2	2	3	4	5	6
Mills, coffee_____no.	1	1	1	2	2	2
Mop handles_____no.	4	6	8	8	10	10
Mortar and pestle, glass, 10-cm_____no.	1	1	1	1	1	1
Mortar and pestle, Wedgwood, 30-cm_____no.	1	1	1	1	1	1
Mortars and pestles, Wedgwood, 8-cm_____no.	1	1	1	1	2	2

* State kind of lamp for which chimneys and wicks are desired.

MISCELLANEOUS—Continued.

ARTICLES.	ALLOWANCE FOR POSTS HAVING OFFICIAL POPULATION OF—					
	100	200	400	600	800	1,000
Mortars and pestles, Wedgwood, 20-cm _____no.	1	1	2	2	3	3
Mouse traps _____no.	2	2	2	2	2	2
Nail puller _____no.	1	1				
Naphthalin, in 5-kilo. boxes _____kilos.	5	5	5	5	5	5
Needle, sailmaker's_____no.	1	1	1	1	1	1
Needle, upholsterer's _____no.	1	1	1	1	1	1
Oil can, with pump, 22-liter _____no.	1	1	1	1	1	1
Pails, milk, with strainer _____no.	1	1	1	2	2	2
Pans, dish _____no.	2	2	2	3	3	3
Pans, dust _____no.	2	2	3	3	4	4
Pans, frying_____no.	1	1	2	2	3	3
Pans, milk _____no.	6	6	8	8	10	10
Pans, muffin_____no.	2	2	3	3	4	4
Pans, sauce _____no.	1	1	1	2	2	2
Paper, filtering, round, 25 cm_____pkg.	2	2	3	3	4	5
Paper, litmus, blue and red, of each_____sheets.	2	2	3	3	4	4
Paper, tarred, in 30-meter rolls_____rolls.	1	1	1	1	1	1
Paper, toilet_____pkgs.	10	15	20	30	40	50
Paper, urinary test, assorted _____pkgs.	1	1	1	1	2	2
Paper, wrapping, blue and white, of each_____qrs.	2	4	6	8	10	12
Paper, wrapping, brown_____qrs.	1	2	3	4	5	6
Pencils, hair, 1 dozen in vial_____doz.	2	3	4	4	5	6
Percolators, glass_____no.	1	1	1	2	2	2
Pickle dishes _____no.	2	2	4	4	5	6
Pill machine _____no.	1	1	1	1	1	1
Pill tile, 12 to 25 cm _____no.	1	1	1	1	1	1
Pipettes, graduated, 5-c. c_____no.	2	2	2	3	3	3
Pitchers, delf, ½-liter _____no.	2	4	4	6	8	10
Pitchers, delf, 1-liter_____no.	2	4	4	6	6	8
Pitchers, sirup, glass_____no.	2	2	3	3	4	4
Plates, dinner _____no.	18	24	36	48	60	72
Potato masher _____no.	1	1	1	1	1	1
Pots, chamber _____no.	2	2	4	4	6	6
Pots, coffee, agate ware or tin_____no.	2	2	2	3	3	3
Pots, tea, agate ware or tin _____no.	2	2	2	3	3	3
Pots, watering_____no.	1	1	1	1	1	1
Prescription file _____no.	1	1	1	1	1	1
Pus basins_____no.	1	1	1	2	2	2
Razor _____no.	1	1	1	1	1	1
Razor strop _____no.	1	1	1	1	1	1
Retort stand _____no.	1	1	1	1	1	1
Rolling-pin _____no.	1	1	1	1	1	1
Saltcellars, glass_____no.	8	8	10	10	12	15
Sapolio _____kilos.	3	4	5	7	10	12
Saucers _____no.	18	24	36	48	60	72
Saw, butcher's_____no.	1	1	1	1	1	1
Saw, hand _____no.	1	1				
Scales and weights, apothecary's_____no.	1	1	1	1	1	1
Scales and weights, balance, in glass case _____no.	1	1	1	1	1	1
Scales and weights, grocer's_____no.	1	1	1	1	1	1
Scales and weights, platform_____no.	1	1	1	1	1	1
Scoops_____no.	1	1	1	2	2	2

MISCELLANEOUS—Continued.

ARTICLES.		Allowance for Posts having Official Population of—				
		100	200	400	600	800	1,000
Screw-drivers, large and small, of each	no.	1	1				
Settees for porch or hall	no.	1	1	2	2	3	3
Shaving brush	no.	1	1	1	1	1	1
Shears	no.	2	2	2	2	2	2
Sickle	no.	1	1	1	1	1	1
Sieves, flour	no.	1	1	1	2	2	2
Skeleton, in cabinet	no.			1	1	1	1
Skimmers	no.	1	1	1	2	2	2
Spatulas, 15-cm	no.	1	1	2	2	2	2
Spatulas, 7-cm	no.	1	1	2	2	2	2
Sponges, bath, large	no.	2	2	2	3	4	4
Spoons, basting, agate ware or tinned iron	no.	2	2	2	2	3	3
Spoons, table, common. (See par. 51.)	no.						
Spoons, table, silver plated. (See par. 51.)	no.	18	24	36	48	56	72
Spoons, tea, common. (See par. 51.)	no.						
Spoons, tea, silver plated. (See par. 51.)	no.	18	24	36	48	56	72
Steels	no.	1	1	1	1	2	2
Stencil, with outfit, for marking hospital clothing	no.	1	1	1	1	1	1
Stove, coal oil, if required	no.	1	1	1	1	1	1
Stove blacking	papers.	6	10	10	20	20	25
Suppository mold	no.	1	1	1	1	1	1
Syringes, penis, glass, in case	no.	30	42	60	72	96	96
Tablet machine, with 200 and 324 mgm. dies	no.	1	1	1	1	1	1
Talcum (French chalk), 1-kilo. packages	kilos.	2	2	2	2	2	2
Tape measures, linen, 1-meter	no.	1	1	1	2	2	2
Test tubes, assorted	no.	12	12	18	18	24	24
Test tubes, stand for	no.	1	1	1	1	1	1
Thermometers, one for each ward	no.						
Tools, chest of	no.			1	1	1	1
Trays, antiseptic	no.	1	1	1	1	2	2
Trays, butler's	no.	2	2	4	4	6	8
Trays, bed, with legs	no.	2	2	4	6	8	8
Trimmer, lamp	no.	1	1	1	1	1	1
Trowel, garden	no.	1	1	1	1	1	1
Tubing, glass, assorted	kilos.	½	⅓	½	1	1	1
Tubing, rubber	meters.	2	2	3	3	4	4
Tumblers, glass	no.	24	36	36	50	60	84
Twine, fine and coarse, of each	gms.	30	30	45	45	60	60
Twine boxes	no.	2	2	2	2	2	2
Urinals, delf or agate ware	no.	4	4	6	6	8	8
Urinometers	no.	1	1	1	2	2	2
Vials, 50 in box, two 180-c. c., twelve 120-c. c., eighteen 60-c. c., twelve 30-c. c., six 15-c. c	boxes.	10	15	20	25	30	35
Vials, 4-c. c	doz.	2	3	4	5	6	7
Washtubs. (See par. 32.)	no.	1	1	1	1	2	2

29

COMPOSITION OF TABLETS.

The words pills, tablets, and trochisci are used synonymously throughout the Supply Table. Compound tablets which are not official and are referred to by these names have the following composition:

ALOINI PILULÆ COMPOSITÆ.

Aloinum	mgms.	8
Podophylli resina	mgms.	8
Belladonnæ fol. ext. alc	mgms.	8
Strychnina	mgms.	0.8
Oleoresina capsici	mgms.	2.7

ANTISEPTIC.

Hydrargyri chloridum corr	mgms.	500
Ammonii chloridum	mgms.	475
One tablet to one-half liter of water makes a 1-to-1000 solution.		

COPAIBÆ PILULÆ COMPOSITÆ.

Copaiba	mgms.	100
Resina guaiaci	mgms.	24
Ferri citras	mgms.	24
Oleoresina cubebæ	mgms.	40

FERRI PILULÆ COMPOSITÆ.

Ferri pyrophosphas	mgms.	65
Quininæ sulphas	mgms.	32
Strychninæ sulphas	mgm.	1

HYDRARG. CHL. MITE CUM. SODIO BICARB.

Hydrargyri chl. mite	mgms.	32
Sodii bicarb	mgms.	65

HYOSCYAMI PILULÆ COMPOSITÆ.

Extractum hyoscyami	mgms.	65
Camphora	mgms.	65
Oleoresina capsici	mgms.	3
Morphinæ acetas	mgms.	3

LINIMENTUM RUBEFACIENS.

Camphora	mgms.	500
Capsicum	mgms.	500
Ext. belladonnæ fol. alc	mgms.	500
Dissolve one tablet in 30 c. c. of alcohol.		

MISTURA GLYCYRRHIZÆ COMPOSITA.

Extractum glycyrrhizæ	mgms.	6
Camphora	mgms.	2.5
Acidum benzoicum	mgms.	2.5
Opium	mgms.	2.5
Antimonii et pot. tartras	mgm.	1
Oleum anisi	mgms.	2.5
Each tablet is the practical equivalent of 4 c. c. of brown mixture.		

PILULÆ CAMPHORÆ ET OPII.

Camphora	mgms.	130
Opium	mgms.	65

PILULÆ CARMINATIVÆ.

Morphinæ sulphas	mgms.	0.8
Camphora	mgms.	16
Extractum rhei	mgms.	32
Sodii carbonas exsic	mgms.	100
Oleoresina capsici	mgms.	2.7
Oleum menthæ piperitæ	mgms.	5

SODII BICARB. ET MENTHÆ PIP.

Sodii bicarbonas	mgms.	258
Ammonii carbonas	mgms.	16
Oleum menthæ piperitæ	mgms.	5

BOTTLES AND JARS CONTAINED IN DISPENSING SET.

TINCTURE BOTTLES.

1-liter	no.	11
500-c. c	no.	9
250-c. c	no.	21
125-c. c	no.	6
60-c. c	no.	18

TINCTURE BOTTLES, BLUE.

125-c. c	no.	2

STEEPLE-TOP JARS.

250-gm	no.	10

SALT-MOUTH BOTTLES.

500-gm	no.	9
250-gm	no.	28
125-gm	no.	22
60-gm	no.	23

SALT-MOUTH BOTTLES, BLUE.

60-gm	no.	4

TOTAL.

Bottles	no.	153
Jars	no.	10

Contents in detail of the cases, etc., to which reference is made in the Supply Table.

APPARATUS—COMPRESSED AIR.

CONTENTS.				
Air container, with gauge _____no.	1	Davidson's sprays, in set, viz :		
Force pump _____no.	1	Atomizer tubes, h. r _____no.	3
Tubing, thick rubber, silk covered, con-		Bottles, with h. r. caps_____no.	3
necting container with cut-off_____meters.	2. 4	Cut-off, metal _____no.	1
Tubing, thick rubber, connecting con-		Stand for bottles _____no.	1
tainer with force pump _____meters.	1. 2	Tube connector, h. r_____no.	1
		Tube, wires for cleaning_____no.	2

APPARATUS—RESTRAINT.

CONTENTS.				
Anklets _____pair.	1	Strap, bed, as per circular _____no.	1
Keys to lock buckles _____no.	5	Strap, waist_____no.	1
Muff, leather_____no.	1	Wristlets _____pair.	1

In wooden box, with handle and lock.

APPARATUS—SPRAY PRODUCING (Rumbold's, for Petrolatum.)

CONTENTS.				
Air bulb, soft rubber _____no.	1	Speculum, nasal, adjustable blades _____no.	1
Mirror, hinged, 3 glasses_____no.	1	Spray producers, metal. (Nos. 1, 2, 4, 5) ____no.	4
		Tongue depressor, 3 blades _____no.	1

CASE—ASPIRATING.

CONTENTS.				
Needles, aspirating _____no.	3	Tube, metallic, with extra wires _____no.	1
Obturator, blunt, for cannula _____no.	1	Tubing attachments _____no.	4
Pump _____no.	1	Tubing, rubber _____pieces.	3
Tube, double current, metal, with rubber stopper_no.	1	Trocar and cannula, with stopcock_____no.	1

In morocco case.

CASE—CAPITAL OPERATING.

Two patterns of cases under this name have been issued, and will be referred to hereafter as Nos. 1 and 2, in accordance with the dates of issue. The contents are essentially the same, but they may be readily distinguished by No. 1 being a narrow, thick case, containing a leaden mallet, while No. 2, which was a part of most of the late personal sets, is a wide, flat case, and does not contain a mallet.

CAPITAL OPERATING CASE, No. 1.

CONTENTS.				
Catling, long_____no.	1	Forceps, artery, fenestrated, spring catch _____no.	1
Catling, small _____no.	1	Forceps, bone, gouge _____no.	1
Chisel _____no	1	Forceps, bone, long, slightly bent_____no.	1
Drills, with one handle _____no.	4	Forceps, bone, long, angled _____no.	1
Elevator and raspatory, combined_____no.	1	Forceps, sequestrum_____no.	1
		Gouge_____no.	1

CASE—CAPITAL OPERATING—Continued.

CAPITAL OPERATING CASE, No. 1—Continued.

Contents.

Hook, double	no.	1	Saw, Hey's	no.	1
Knife, amputating, long	no.	1	Saw, metacarpal	no.	1
Knife, amputating, medium	no.	1	Scalpels	no.	3
Knife, cartilage	no.	1	Scissors, straight	no.	1
Ligature, silk	gms.	5	Tenaculum	no.	1
Mallet, leaden	no.	1	Tourniquet, screw	no.	1
Needle, aneurism, handle and 3 tips	no.	1	Trephine, brush for	no.	1
Needle, key, artery	no.	1	Trephine, conical	no.	1
Needles, surgeon's	no.	12	Trephine, crown	no.	1
Retractors	no.	2	Trephine, handle for	no.	1
Saw, bow, 2 blades	no.	1	Wax	piece.	1
Saw, chain	no.	1			

In mahogany case, with leather pouch.

CAPITAL OPERATING CASE, No. 2.

Contents.

Bistoury, straight	no.	1	Needle, key, artery	no.	1
Catling, long	no.	1	Needles, surgeon's	no.	12
Catling, small	no.	1	Raspatory	no.	1
Chisel	no.	1	Razor	no.	1
Drills, with one handle	no.	4	Retractors	no.	2
Elevator	no.	1	Saw, bow, 2 blades	no.	1
Forceps, artery, bulbous, slide catch	no.	1	Saw, chain	no.	1
Forceps, bone, gouge, curved	no.	1	Saw, Hey's	no.	1
Forceps, bone, gouge, straight	no.	1	Saw, movable back	no.	1
Forceps, bone, long	no.	1	Scalpels	no.	3
Forceps, lithotomy	no.	1	Scissors, straight	no.	1
Forceps, sequestrum	no.	1	Tenaculum	no.	2
Gouge	no.	1	Tourniquet, screw, with pad	no.	1
Knife, amputating, long	no.	1	Trephine, brush for	no.	1
Knife, amputating, medium	no.	1	Trephine, conical	no.	2
Knife, cartilage	no.	1	Trephine, handle for	no.	1
Ligature, silk	gms.	5	Trocar and cannula, straight	no.	1
Needle, aneurism, handle and 3 tips	no.	1	Wax	piece.	1

In mahogany case, with leather pouch.

CASE—DENTAL.

Contents.

Burnishers (Nos. 3, 29, 36)	no.	3	Gutta-percha	gms.	30
Chisels (Nos. 77, 135)	no.	2	Handles for instruments	no.	6
Explorer (No. 5)	no.	1	Hone	no.	1
Excavators (Nos. 10, 14, 16, 21, 41, 82, 86, 141, 143, 145)	no.	10	Mirror	no.	1
			Paper, bibulous	sheets.	6
Files (2 each of Nos. 00, 0, 1)	no.	6	Scaler (No. 3)	no.	1
Forceps, college	no.	1	Spatula (No. 1)	no.	1

In small morocco case.

CASE—EMERGENCY.

TABLETS IN 15-C C. BOTTLES.			Quininæ sulphas	mgms.	200
Acetanilidum	mgms.	200	Sulphonal	mgm.	324
Acidum tannicum	mgms.	324	HYPODERMIC TABLETS, IN TUBES.		
Aconiti tinctura	c. c.	0.1	Apomorphinæ hydrochloras*	mgms.	6
Aloini composita			Atropinæ sulphas*	mgms.	0.65
Antipyrinum	mgms.	324	Cocainæ hydrochloras	mgms.	10
Antiseptic			Digitalinum *	mgms.	1
Bismuthi subnitras	mgms.	324	Morphinæ sulphas *	mgms.	8
Carminative			Nitroglycerinum	mgms.	0.65
Catharticæ composite			Quininæ hydrochloras	mgms.	32
Chloral	mgms.	324	Strychninæ sulphas	mgms.	1
Digitalis tinctura	c. c.	0.3			
Ergotinum	mgms.	130	INSTRUMENTS.		
Hydrargyrum chl. mite cum sodio bicarb			Bistoury, curved and straight, of each	no.	1
Ipecacuanha et opium			Forceps, hæmostatic	no.	1
Morphinæ sulphas	mgms.	8	Ligature, silk	gm.	1
Opii tinctura camphorata	c. c.	0.4	Needles, surgical	no.	6
Phenacetinum	mgms.	324	Plaster, isinglass	roll.	1
Potassii bromidum	mgms.	324	Scissors, straight	no.	1

Syringe, hypodermic	no.	1
Thermometer, clinical	no.	1

* Tablets marked thus are in the hypodermic syringe case.

CASE—EYE AND EAR.

This list does not correspond to the contents of all eye and ear cases ; discrepancies should be noted.

CONTENTS.				
Bottles, g. s., &c. c.	no.	2	Needle, curved	no.	1
Catheter, eustachian, h. r	no.	1	Needle, stop, curved	no.	1
Curette	no.	1	Needle, stop, straight	no.	1
Cystotome and scoop	no.	1	Needle, straight	no.	1
Director, lachrymal	no.	1	Needles, fine	no.	6
Forceps, angular, for ear	no.	1	Ophthalmoscope	no.	1
Forceps, cilia	no.	1	Optometer (Thomson's)	no.	1
Forceps, fixation	no.	1	Probes, lachrymal, double, silver	no.	4
Forceps, iridectomy, angular	no.	1	Scalpel	no.	1
Forceps, iridectomy, curved	no.	1	Scissors, curved on the flat	no.	1
Forceps, iridectomy, straight	no.	1	Scissors, iris (Noyes's), on handle	no.	1
Hook, blunt	no.	1	Scissors, strabismus	no.	1
Hook, blunt, curved shank	no.	1	Scissors, straight	no.	1
Hook, double	no.	1	Scoop and hook, metal handle	no.	1
Hook, strabismus	no.	2	Silk, fine	gm.	1
Keratome, angular	no.	2	Speculum, ear, in nest	no.	3
Knife (Beer's), cataract	no.	1	Speculum, eye, stop	no.	1
Knife (Graefe's), linear	no.	1	Speculum, eye, stop (Graefe's)	no.	1
Knife, iris	no.	1	Spoon, lens, h. r	no.	1
Knife, iris, double-edge	no.	1	Spoon, lens, fenestrated	no.	1
Lid holder, large and small	no.	2	Spud, Dix's	no.	1
Lid holder, hard rubber	no.	1	Styles, lachrymal, silver	no.	2
Mirror, laryngeal	no.	2	Syringe (Anel's), with 3 tips	no.	1
Mirror, laryngoscopic, with head band	no.	1	Wax	piece.	1

In mahogany case, with leather pouch.

CASE—FIELD.*

In wooden case, with leather pouch and sling strap with buckle and snap hooks.

CONTENTS.					
Bistoury, curved	no.	1	Ligature, silk	gms.	3
Catheter, silver, jointed	no.	1	Needles, surgeon's	no.	12
Director and aneurism needle	no.	1	Probe (Nélaton's)	no.	1
Forceps, artery and needle, combined	no.	1	Saw blade, movable back	no.	1
Forceps, bone	no.	1	Saw blade, handle	no.	1
Forceps, bullet	no.	1	Scalpel	no.	1
Forceps, dressing	no.	1	Scissors, straight	no.	1
Knife, amputating, blade	no.	1	Serrefines (Langenbeck's)	no.	4
Knife, amputating, handle	no.	1	Tenaculum	no.	1
			Wax	piece.	1

* This is the case recently issued as "surgeon's field case."

CASE—FIELD OPERATING.

This list does not correspond to the contents of all field operating cases; discrepancies should be noted.

CONTENTS.					
Bistoury, curved	no.	1	Needle, key, artery	no.	1
Bistoury, curved, probe-pointed	no.	1	Needles, surgeon's	no.	12
Bistoury, straight	no.	2	Probe, bullet, long	no.	1
Catheters, silver, Nos. 3, 6, and 9	no.	3	Probe (Nélaton's)	no.	1
Catling, long	no.	1	Razor	no.	1
Catling, medium	no.	1	Retractors	no.	2
Director	no.	1	Saw, bow, 2 blades	no.	1
Elevator	no.	1	Saw, chain	no.	1
Elevator and raspatory, combined	no.	1	Saw, Hey's	no.	1
Forceps, artery, spring	no.	1	Saw, metacarpal	no.	1
Forceps, bone, curved	no.	1	Scalpel	no.	1
Forceps, bullet	no.	1	Scissors, angular	no.	1
Forceps, dissecting	no.	1	Scissors, straight	no.	1
Forceps, dressing	no.	1	Sounds, steel, silvered, double curve, Nos. 1-2,		
Forceps, sequestrum	no.	1	3-4, 5-6, 7-8, 9-10, 11-12	no.	6
Knife, amputating, long	no.	1	Tenaculum	no.	1
Knife, amputating, medium	no.	1	Tourniquet, screw, with pad	no.	1
Knife, hernia	no.	1	Trephine, brush for	no.	1
Ligature, silk	gms.	5	Trephine, conical, and handle	no.	1
Needle, aneurism, handle and 3 tips	no.	1	Trocar and cannula, curved	no.	1
			Wax	piece.	1

In mahogany case, with leather pouch.

CASE—FORCEPS, HÆMOSTATIC.

CONTENTS.					
Halstead's straight	no.	1	Tait's long grip	no.	1
Halstead's curved	no.	1	Tait's short grip	no.	1
Jones's angular	no.	1	Thornton's T	no.	1
Jones's straight	no.	1	Wood's (Péan's) large	no.	2
Little's fenestrated	no.	1	Wood's (Péan's) small	no.	2

In morocco case.

34

CASE—GENITO-URETHRAL.

Contents.

Bougies à boule (Otis's), metal, nickel-plated,
   Nos. 11, 14, 17, 21, 26, 30 _____no.   6
Catheter, double current, silver _____no.   1
Catheter, grooved and tunneled (Gouley's),
   with stylet _____no.   1
Catheter and staff, grooved and tunneled
   (Gouley's), with stylet _____no.   1
Urin de Florence_____no.   1
Dilator (Thompson's), modified by Gouley ____no.   1
Director, silver (Gouley's) _____no.   1

Forceps, urethral (Thompson's) _____no.   1
Gauge, steel (American and French) _____no.   1
Gauges, pasteboard (American and French) ____no.   2
Guides, whalebone (Gouley's) _____no.   12
Guides, whalebone (Otis's) _____no.   2
Knife, beaked (Gouley's) _____no.   1
Sounds, set of 4, fitting one handle _____set.   1
Sounds, tunneled (Gouley's) _____no.   3
Tenaculum (Gouley's) _____no.   1
Urethrotome, dilating (Gouley's), with two
   tunneled tips _____no.   1

In rosewood case.

CASE—GENITO-URINARY.

Contents.

Bistoury for meatus (Otis's) _____no.   1
Bougies à boule (Otis's), metal, nickel-plated,
   Nos. 8 to 40, inclusive _____no.   33
Endoscopes (Otis's, h. r.), Nos. 22, 26, and 32 __no.   3
Gauge (Otis's), steel _____no.   1
Guides (Otis's), whalebone _____no.   2
Sounds (Otis's), short-beaked, steel, nickel-
   plated, Nos. 20 to 40, inclusive _____no.   21

Urethrometer (Otis's), hinged _____no.   1
Urethrometer, rubber covers for _____no.   12
Urethrotome, Maisonneuve's, No. 8, Otis's
   gauge, with two blades, two filiform bougies
   and one extra tunneled tip for whalebone
   guide _____no.   1
Urethrotome, dilating (Otis's), straight, with
   two blades _____no.   1

In mahogany case.

CASE—URETHRAL.

But few of these have been issued. It is essentially the same as the genito-urinary case, but the arrangement and contents are somewhat different.

Contents.

Bougies à boule (Otis's), metal, nickel-plated,
   Nos. 8 to 46, inclusive _____no.   39
Catheter syringe, prostatic _____no.   1
Gauge, steel _____no.   1
Sounds (Otis's), short-beaked, steel, nickel-
   plated, Nos. 21 to 46, inclusive _____no.   26

Urethrometer (Otis's), spring _____no.   1
Urethrometer, rubber covers for _____no.   12
Urethrotome, dilating (Otis's), straight, with
   two blades _____no.   1

In rosewood case, with lock.

CASE—MINOR OPERATING.

Contents.

Bistoury, curved _____no.   1
Bistoury, curved, probe-pointed _____no.   1
Bistoury, straight _____no.   2
Cannula (Bellocq's) _____no.   1
Catheter, prostatic, silver _____no.   1
Catheters, silver, Nos. 3, 6, and 9 _____no.   3
Director _____no.   1
Ecraseur, wire, two tips_____no.   1
Forceps, artery, fenestrated, slide catch ____no.   1
Forceps, bullet_____no.   1

Forceps, dissecting _____no.   1
Forceps, dressing _____no.   1
Forceps, œsophageal_____no.   1
Forceps, tracheotomy (Trousseau's) _____no.   1
Knife, amputating _____no.   1
Knife, hernia_____no.   1
Ligature, silk_____gms.   5
Needle, artery, with four tips_____no.   1
Needle, key, artery_____no.   1
Needles, surgeon's_____no.   12
Pliers, wire-cutting, small_____no.   1

CASE—MINOR OPERATING—Continued.

Contents.

Probang, œsophageal	no. 1
Probe (Nélaton's)	no. 1
Probe (Sayre's) vertebrated	no. 1
Scalpels	no. 2
Scissors, angular	no. 1
Scissors, curved	no. 1
Scissors, straight	no. 1
Serrefines	no. 6
Sound, small	no. 1
Sounds, steel, silvered, double-curve, Nos. 1-2, 3-4, 5-6, 7-8, 9-10, 11-12	no. 6
Staff, grooved, large	no. 1
Staff, grooved, medium	no. 1
Staff (Syme's)	no. 1
Tenaculum	no. 1
Tonsillotome	no. 1
Trocar and cannula, curved	no. 1
Tubes, tracheotomy, double	no. 2
Wax	piece. 1

In brass-bound mahogany case, with leather pouch.

CASE—OBSTETRICAL AND GYNECOLOGICAL.

Contents.

Blunt hook and crotchet, guarded	no. 1
Bottle, g. s. and g. c., for Little's saline mixture	no. 1
Bottle, g. s. and g. c., for styptic	no. 1
Bottle, g. s. and g. c., for ergot	no. 1
Catheter (Sims's), sigmoid, metal	no. 1
Cephalotribe (craniotomy forceps)	no. 1
Dilators (Barnes's), with stopcocks, etc.	no. 3
Dilator, uterine, small	no. 1
Elevator, uterine (Sims's), with two points	no. 1
Forceps, long (Wallace's)	no. 1
Forceps, placenta (Loomis's)	no. 1
Forceps, short (Brickell's)	no. 1
Funis clamp (Pulling's)	no. 1
Perforator (Thomas's)	no. 1
Probe, uterine, silver, with silver applicator, set-screw handle, and sponge tent expeller	no. 1
Scarifier (Buttles's)	no. 1
Scissors, uterine, curved on the flat	no. 1
Sound, folding (Simpson's)	no. 1
Speculum, vaginal and anal, combined	no. 1
Suppository tube, intra-uterine, h. r.	no. 1
Syringe, rubber, self-injecting	no. 1
Tampon, small	no. 1
Tenaculum (Nott's)	set. 1
Transfusion set (Fryer's) *	no. 1
Vectis, with handle	no. 1

In leather trunk case, with handles and lock.

* With directions for use, and consisting of a rubber tube with two bulbs, a glass receiver, and giver's and receiver's cannulæ.

CASE—POCKET, ASEPTIC.

Contents.

Bistoury, curved	no. 1
Bistoury, curved, probe-pointed	no. 1
Bistoury, straight	no. 1
Catheter, jointed, male and female tips	no. 1
Caustic holder	no. 1
Forceps, needle and fenestrated, artery	no. 1
Forceps, long-jawed	no. 1
Lancet, thumb	no. 1
Ligature, silk	gm. 1
Needle, aneurism	no. 1
Needle, aneurism, and grooved director	no. 1
Needle, exploring	no. 1
Needles, surgeon's	no. 12
Probe (Nélaton's)	no. 1
Probe, silver	no. 1
Scalpel	no. 1
Scissors	no. 1
Tenaculum	no. 1
Tenatome	no. 1
Wax	piece. 1

In leather case, with metal clips and chamois cover.

CASE—POCKET, PERSONAL.

This case was formerly part of the "personal set."

CONTENTS.				
Bistoury, curved	no.	1	Ligature, silk	gm.	1
Bistoury, curved, probe-pointed	no.	1	Needle, aneurism	no.	1
Bistoury, straight	no.	1	Needle, exploring	no.	1
Catheter, jointed, male and female tips	no.	1	Needle, surgeon's	no.	9
Caustic holder	no.	1	Probes	no.	2
Director, grooved	no.	1	Probe (Nélaton's)	no.	1
Forceps, artery, fenestrated	no.	1	Scalpel	no.	1
Forceps, dissecting	no.	1	Scissors	no.	1
Forceps, dressing	no.	1	Tenaculum	no.	1
Lancet, thumb	no.	1	Tenotome	no.	1
			Wax	piece.	1

In leather case, with leather or gutta-percha cover.

CASE—POCKET, POST.

This name will be used when reference is made to the red morocco pocket case with chamois cover issued during the past few years for post use.

The list of contents is the same as that of the aseptic pocket case, but the aneurism and exploring needles, knives, and tenaculum are detachable from the two hard-rubber or ivory handles. Some cases contain a combined needle and fenestrated artery forceps and a hæmostatic forceps, others a plain artery and a dressing forceps.

CASE—POST-MORTEM.

Most of the post-mortem cases now in use are in accordance with the following list:

Blowpipe	no.	1	Knife, amputating, small	no.	1
Chain and hooks	no.	1	Knife, cartilage	no.	1
Chisel	no.	1	Needles (and thread)	no.	2
Costotome chisel	no.	1	Saw	no.	1
Enterotome	no.	1	Scalpels, assorted	no.	3
Forceps, dissecting	no.	1	Scissors, straight	no.	1
Hammer, steel	no.	1	Tenaculum	no.	1
Knife, amputating, large	no.	1			

Handles of saw and of all knives are of ebony; those of costotome, hammer, and tenaculum are of steel. In mahogany box.

DISSECTING CASE.

This case is dropped from the regular list of the Supply Table, as it is practically duplicated by the post-mortem case. Those now on hand will be issued to the smaller posts in lieu of the larger post-mortem case. Its contents are as follows:

Blowpipe	no.	1	Knife, cartilage	no.	1
Chain and hooks	no.	1	Needles (and thread)	no.	2
Chisel	no.	1	Scalpels, assorted	no.	3
Enterotome	no.	1	Scissors, straight	no.	1
Forceps, dissecting	no.	1	Tenaculum	no.	1

In wooden case.

CASE—STOMACH PUMP.

In mahogany case, with lock and key.

CASE—TOOTH EXTRACTING.

In leather-covered case, with lock and double handle.

CASE OF TRIAL LENSES.

BAUSCH & LOMB.

Twenty pairs spherical convex lenses.
Twenty pairs spherical concave lenses, both from 2 to 100 English inches focus. (D. 20–0.35.)
Eleven cylindrical convex lenses.
Eleven cylindrical concave lenses, both from 8.88 to 160 English inches focus. (D. 4. 50–0.25.)
Six prisms, 2°, 3°, 4°, 5°, 8°, 12°.
Five discs, one white and one ground glass, one plain metal, one metal with hole in center, and one metal with stenopaic slit.
Four colored glasses—red, blue, green, and brown.
One graduated trial frame, No. 3, double cell.
One graduated trial frame, No. 2, double cell, adjustable.

In mahogany case, with lock and two keys.

QUEEN.

Twenty pairs spherical convex lenses.
Twenty pairs spherical concave lenses, both from 2 to 48 inches focus.
Eight cylindrical convex lenses.
Eight cylindrical concave lenses, both from 9 to 72 inches focus.
Five prisms, 2°, 3°, 4°, 5°, 8°.
Three metal discs, one plain, one with hole in center, and one with stenopaic slit.
Four colored glasses—red, blue, green, and brown.
One single lens holder.
One trial frame.

In mahogany case, with lock and key.

INHALER AND VAPORIZER.

This consists of a nickel-plated stand, with boiler, spirit lamp, and detachable handle. There are two attachments, a long inhaler and short deodorizer; both have a reservoir holding sponge saturated with the preparation to be vaporized.

MICROSCOPES.

The names of the manufacturer and of the microscope will be noted on all invoices, receipts, and property returns.

The "Universal" Microscope made by the Bausch & Lomb Optical Company is the latest one issued by the Medical Department. It is in two cases, the contents of which are as follows :

MICROSCOPE CASE.		CASE OF MICROSCOPICAL ACCESSORIES.	
Stand, "Universal" -------------no.	1	Microtome ------------------no.	1
Glass stage and slide carrier -----------no.	1	Knife for same, one side flat, in case-----no.	1
Eyepieces, A and C------------------no.	2	Syringe, brass, with four pipes and stopcock, in	
Eyepiece micrometer ---------------no.	1	case---------------------no.	1
Concave and plain mirror -----------no.	1	Turntable, self-centering------------no.	1
Objective, 2-inch -----------------no.	1	Glass slides-----------------doz.	4
Objective, ¾-inch -----------------no.	1	Glass covers----------------gms.	30
Objective, ½-inch -----------------no.	1	Carmine--------------------gms.	15
Objective, 1/12-inch -----------------no.	1	Canada balsam----------------gms.	30
Abbe condenser with iris diaphragm-------no.	1	Balsam bottle----------------no.	1
Double nosepiece -----------------no.	1	Dropping bottle, for oil of cedar--------no.	1
Iris diaphragm, with substage adapter arranged		Gentian violet----------------gms.	4
to take diaphragm or objective ----------no.	1	Bismarck brown---------------gms.	4
Revolving diaphragm ----------------no.	1	Methyl blue-----------------gms.	4
Bull's-eye condenser ---------------no.	1	Fuchsin--------------------gms.	4
Stage forceps -------------------no.	1	Anilino oil-------------------c. c.	60
Camera lucida-------------------no.	1	Paraffin--------------------kilo.	¼
Forceps----------------------no.	1		
Glass covers -------------------no.	6		
Glass slides-------------------no.	6		

In upright cherry wood case, with handle, lock, and extra hook and post fastenings.

In cherry wood case, with handle, lock, and extra hook and post fastenings.

NOTE—

Eyepiece A, 2-inch objective gives about 25 diam. | Eyepiece C, 2-inch objective gives about 50 diam.
Eyepiece A, ¾-inch objective gives about 50 diam. | Eyepiece C, ¾-inch objective gives about 100 diam.
Eyepiece A, ½-inch objective gives about 210 diam. | Eyepiece C, ½-inch objective gives about 420 diam.
Eyepiece A, 1/12-inch objective gives about 570 diam. | Eyepiece C, 1/12-inch objective gives about 1140 diam.

The "Investigator" Microscope, made by the Bausch & Lomb Optical Company, and of which many have been issued, consists of the following :

MICROSCOPE CASE.		CASE OF MICROSCOPICAL ACCESSORIES.	
The contents of this case are the same as those of the Universal Microscope, the stand alone being of a slightly different pattern.		Section cutter, with freezing apparatus --------no.	1
		Razor, large, one side flat, with handle, in case-no.	1
		Syringe, 15-c. c., brass, with four pipes and stop-	
		cock, in case----------------no.	1
		Turntable, self-centering-------------no.	1
		Glass covers----------------gms.	30
		Glass slides-----------------doz.	4
		Carmine--------------------gms.	15
		Canada balsam----------------gms.	30
		Balsam bottle----------------no.	1
		Dropping bottle, for cedar oil ---------no.	1

In cases, etc., as above.

MICROSCOPES—Continued.

A few "Beck's Popular Binocular" microscopes are still in use, and consist of the following in one case, or sometimes in two :

MICROSCOPE.	
Stand ___no.	1
Glass (or brass) stage and slide carrier ___no.	1
Eyepieces ___no.	2
Eyepiece micrometer ___no	1
Concave and plain mirror ___no.	1
Objective, 2-inch ___no.	1
Objective, ¾-inch ___no.	1
Objective, ⅛-inch ___no.	1
Iris diaphragm, with substage adapter, arranged to take diaphragm or objective ___no.	1
Revolving diaphragm ___no.	1
Bull's-eye condenser ___no.	1
Stage forceps ___no.	1
Camera lucida ___no.	1
Forceps ___no.	1
Glass covers ___no.	6
Glass slides ___no.	6

MICROSCOPICAL ACCESSORIES.	
Section cutter with freezing apparatus ___no.	1
Razor, large, one side flat, with handle, in case ___no.	1
Syringe, 15-c. c., brass, with four pipes and stop-cock, in case ___no.	1
Turntable, self-centering ___no.	1
Glass covers ___gms.	30
Glass slides ___doz.	4
Carmine ___gms.	15
Canada balsam ___gms.	30
Balsam bottle ___no.	1

POUCH—HOSPITAL CORPS.

CONTENTS.		
Ammoniæ spiritus aromaticus ___c. c.	30	
Bandages, roller ___no.	4	
Candle, in tin box ___no.	1	
First-aid packet ___no.	1	
Forceps, dressing* ___no.	1	
Iodoform sprinkler ___no.	1	
Jackknife ___no.	1	
Lint, sublimated ___gms.	60	
Needles* ___paper.	1	

Petrolatum, carbolized ___gms.	15	
Pins, common* ___paper.	1	
Pins, safety* ___no.	6	
Plaster, adhesive ___spool.	1	
Scissors* ___no.	1	
Splints, wire ___no.	2	
Sponges, small, in bag ___no.	2	
Thread, linen* ___meters.	18	
Tourniquets, field ___no.	2	
Wool, boracic ___gms.	60	

POUCH—ORDERLY.

CONTENTS.		
Ammoniæ spiritus aromaticus ___c. c.	30	
Bandages, roller ___no.	2	
Basin, pus ___no.	1	
Case, medicine, with tablets † ___no.	1	
Catheter, elastic (No. 8) ___no.	1	
Chloroformum ___c. c.	125	
First-aid packet ___no.	1	
Glass, medicine ___no.	1	
Lint, sublimated ___gms.	60	

Petrolatum, carbolized ___gms.	15	
Pins, common ___paper.	1	
Pins, safety ___no.	6	
Scissors, medium ___no.	1	
Sponges, small, in bag ___no.	2	
Syringe, hypodermic ___no.	1	
Tags, diagnosis, with pencil ___book.	1	
Tourniquet, Esmarch's ___no.	1	
Wool, boracic ___gms.	60	

*Articles marked thus are contained in special case.

† The six 15-c. c. bottles in this case contain the following tablets :

Acetanilidum ___mgms. ___200		Catharticæ compositæ ___	
Antiseptic ___		Mistura glycyrrhizæ comp ___	
Carminativm ___		Quininæ sulphas ___mgms. ___200	

SURGICAL PUMP.

Allen's Surgical Pump, No. 12, will in future be supplied, and consists of the following outfit :

CONTENTS.					
Bottles, g. s	no.	2	Dilator, uterine, small	no.	1
Bottles (vials)	no.	2	Dilator, uterine, silk covers for	no.	4
Catheter and connector	no.	1	Needles, aspirating	no.	4
Clamp attachment	no.	1	Pipe, breast (nipple glass)	no.	1
Cock, two-way, rubber, for injecting	no.	1	Pipes, syringe (ear, post nasal, vaginal, rectal,		
Connector tube	no.	1	and uterine)	no.	5
Connectors with cut-offs	no.	3	Pump, 9 cm. and tube	no.	1
Couplings, "Universal"	no.	2	Pump, extra tube for	no.	1
Cupper, uterine, metal	no.	1	Tampons	no.	2
Cupping glasses	no.	5	Tampons, extra bags for	no.	4
Dilator, uterine, large	no.	1	Trocar, dome	no.	1
			Tube, stomach and connector	no.	1

In leather bag, with lock and key, and directions for use. Those heretofore issued are of two or three different patterns, and do not exactly correspond to the above list.

SYRINGE—HYPODERMIC.

These syringes as now issued have as accessories, besides two needles and extra wires, one tube of each of the following hypodermic tablets :

Apomorphinæ hydrochloras	mgms.	6	Digitalinum	mgms.	1
Atrophinæ sulphas	mgms.	0.65	Morphinæ sulphas	mgms.	8

The needles and wires are expendable.

THERMO-CAUTERY, PAQUELIN'S.

An improved pattern has recently been adopted. The contents are the same except that the combustion chamber or lamp is omitted, the modified reservoir for hydrocarbon rendering it unnecessary.

CONTENTS.					
Apparatus, double bulb, for supplying air	no.	1	Handle, cannulated, ebony	no.	1
Cautery button	no.	1	Reservoir for hydrocarbon, nickel plated	no.	1
Cautery knife	no.	1	Tube, lengthening	no.	1
Combustion chamber (lamp), nickel plated	no.	1	Tube, rubber	no.	1

In morocco case.

TYPEWRITER.

The typewriting machine, as issued, has the following outfit :

Impression strips (extra)	no.	2	Ribbon shield (extra)	no.	1
Key for mainspring	no.	1	Screw-driver	no.	1
Oil can	no.	1	Spools, for ribbons	pairs.	2
Oil	bott.	1	Type-wheel, large and small capitals	no.	1
Ribbon, copying, indelible	no.	1	Type-wheel, large Roman	no.	1
Ribbon, record, black	no.	1	Type-wheel, small Roman	no.	1

With printed circular of instructions.

VISION-TEST SET.

This set contains—

1. A set of three test cards for use at distances of 13, 16½, and 20 feet, respectively, bearing the test characters authorized by Greenleaf's Epitome of Tripler's Manual, p. 38.

2. A simple optometer consisting of two lenses, one of 4-inch and the other of 10-inch focal length; a brass holder with graduated bar and sliding test-type holder; six test-type cards, numbered 1, for the measurement of defects of refraction and accommodation, and six test-type cards, numbered 2, for the measurement of astigmatism.

3. A set of test wools for the detection of color blindness, consisting of three larger skeins of "test colors" (one pale green, one rose color, called purple, and one bright red); and one hundred and forty-four small skeins of "confusion colors," as follows:

Of pure gray, four shades, two skeins of each.

Of the colors named below, eight shades, one skein of each, all wrapped in a piece of muslin 1 meter square.

Hair-brown.	Orange.	Blue, No. 1.
Lion-brown.	Yellow.	Blue, No. 2.
Olive-brown.	Yellow-green.	Violet.
Wood-brown.	Olive-green.	Purple, No. 1 (Rose Victoria).
Pearl-gray.	Green.	Purple, No. 2.
Scarlet.	Blue-green.	

4. A small paper box in which to keep the extra lens and the twelve test-type cards.
5. A pamphlet of directions for using the vision-test set.
6. A painted tin box containing all the foregoing.

The cases named in the following list, viz. amputating, exsecting, general operating, and trephining, formed the "personal set" issued to medical officers prior to 1868. Upon the adoption in the latter year of the personal set until recently issued individually to medical officers the former cases were transferred to hospitals as post cases of instruments, and a considerable number are still in use.

AMPUTATING CASE.

CONTENTS.				
Catling, long ____no.	1	Ligature silk ____gms.	2
Catling, small ____no.	1	Needle, aneurism ____no.	1
Forceps, artery, spring-catch ____no.	1	Needles, surgeon's ____no.	12
Forceps, bone (nippers) ____no.	1	Saw, bow, two blades ____no.	1
Knife, amputating, long ____no.	1	Saw, metacarpal ____no.	1
Knife, amputating, medium ____no.	1	Scalpel ____no.	1
Knife, amputating, small ____no.	1	Tenaculum ____no.	1
		Tourniquet, screw, with pad ____no.	1
		Wax ____piece.	1

In mahogany case.

EXSECTING CASE.

CONTENTS.				
Chisel ____no.	1	Forceps, sequestrum ____no.	1
Ecraseur, chain ____no.	1	Gouge ____no.	1
Forceps, bone, gouge ____no.	2	Knife, lenticular ____no.	1
Forceps, bone, long ____no.	1	Retractors ____no.	2
		Saw, chain ____no.	1
		Trephine ____no.	1

In mahogany case, with gutta-percha cover.

GENERAL OPERATING CASE.

This set consists of two mahogany boxes with locks and key, carried in a leather or heavy gutta-percha pouch, and containing the following :

Box No. 1.				
Bistoury, curved	no.	1	Needle, key, artery	no.	1
Bistoury, curved, probe-pointed	no.	1	Needles surgeon's	no.	12
Bistoury, straight	no.	1	Saw, movable back	no.	1
Catling	no.	1	Scissors, curved	no.	1
Forceps, bullet	no.	1	Scissors, straight	no.	1
Forceps, dissecting	no.	1	Scalpels	no.	3
Forceps, dressing, curved	no.	1	Tenaculum	no.	1
Forceps, œsophageal	no.	1	Tourniquet, field	no.	1
Hook, double	no.	1	Trocar and cannula, straight	no.	1
Knife, amputating, small	no.	1	Box No. 2.		
Knife, hernia	no.	1	Catheters, metallic	no.	3
Needle, aneurism, handle and four tips	no.	1	Sounds, metallic, double-curve	no.	6
Needle, cataract	no.	1			

TREPHINING CASE.

Contents.					
Elevator	no.	1	Trephine, brush for	no.	2
Saw (Hey's)	no.	1	Trephine, conical	no.	1
Scalpel and raspatory	no.	1	Trephine, handle for	no.	1

In small mahogany box.

CHEMICAL SET.

CHEMICALS.

Acid, arsenous As_2O_3	grams.	50	Potassium ferrocyanid, $K_4Fe(CN)_6 3H_2O$		
Acid, oxalic, $H_2C_2O_4 2H_2O$	grams.	100		grams.	25
Alcohol, ethylic, abs. C_2H_5OH	grams.	100	Potassium hydrate, KOH	grams.	200
Ammonium molybdate $(NH_4)_2MoO_4$	grams.	60	Potassium sulphocyanate, $KSCN$	grams.	50
Anilin $C_6H_5NH_2$	grams.	50	Sodium phosphate, dry, Na_2HPO_4	grams.	50
Barium chlorid, $BaCl_2 2H_2O$	grams.	50	Sodium hydrato, $NaOH$	grams.	200
Calcium carbonate, $CaCo_3$	grams.	50	Sodium thiosulphate, $Na_2S_2O_3 5H_2O$	grams.	100
Calcium chlorid, $CaCl_2$	grams.	50	Stannous chlorid, $SnCl_2 2H_2O$	grams.	50
Ferrous sulfid FeS	grains.	100	Uranic nitrate, $UO_2(NO_3)_2 6H_2O$	grams.	50
Potassium dichromate, $K_2Cr_2O_7$	grams.	100	Methyl orange, $HC_{14}H_{14}N_3SO_3$	grams.	10
Potassium cyanid, KCN	grams.	50	Naphthylamine, $C_{10}H_7NH_2$	grams.	5
Potassium ferricyanid, $K_6Fe(CN)_{12}$	grams.	25	Phenolphthalein, $C_{20}H_{14}O_4$	grams.	10

APPARATUS.

Beakers, 100–200 c. c.	no.	6	Crucibles, porcelain, conical	no.	4
Bottles, g. s. n. m. 50, 100, 200 c. c.	no.	24	Filters, cut, white (in packs of 100)	pkgs.	3
Burette	no.	2	Flasks, flat bottomed, with lip	no.	6
Burette clips	no.	4	Flasks, round bottomed, long neck	no.	2
Capsules, porcelain, nest of six	nest.	1	Flasks, Schuster's, stoppered	no.	6
Capsules, porcelain, 100-c. c.	no.	6	Forceps, small	no.	1
Capsules, porcelain, 250-c. c.	no.	3	Funnel tubes	no.	2
Corks, india rubber, perforated	doz.	1	Funnels, glass	no.	2

APPARATUS—Continued.

Glasses, Nessler, 50-c. c	no.	6	Spatulas or spoons, porcelain	no.	2
Pipe, block tin, 9-mm., for condensing distilled water	meters.	6	Still, copper, 2-liter	no.	1
			Stopcocks for rubber tubing	no.	2
Pipettes, 10-c. c	no.	2	Test glasses, footed	no.	12
Pipettes, 25-c. c	no.	1	Tubes, Ca Cl	no.	2
Pipettes, 10-c. c., graduated	no.	1	Tubes, U	no.	3
Platinum crucible, 30-c. c	no.	1	Wash bottle	no.	1
Retorts, 1-liter, stoppered	no.	2	Watch glasses	no.	6
Rods, glass	no.	12	Water bath for drying	no.	1

MISCELLANEOUS.

Aluminium foil	grams.	15	Platinum foil	sq. cm.	20
Copper foil	grams.	25	Wire gauze	sq. cm.	50
Glass, blue	sq. cm.	9	Zinc foil	sq. cm.	20
Iron wire	grams.	50	Zinc, granulated	grams.	100

BACTERIOLOGICAL SET.

Apparatus, filling, and stand	no.	1	Platinum wire, medium, 10-cm	pieces.	6
Bath, water, copper	no.	1	Regulator, gas (Reichert's)	no.	1
Bath, tripod for	no.	1	Sterilizer, hot-air, cm. 38 x 28 x 25.5	no.	1
Burner, stand for	no.	1	Stoppers, solid rubber, assorted	kilo.	1.4
Dishes, double (Petri's)	no.	12	Syringe, sterilizable (Koch's), 1-c. c	no.	1
Filters (Pasteur's), mounted in flask	no.	2	Test measures, footed, 10-c. c	no.	1
Flasks (Erlenmeyer's), 236-c. c	no.	12	Test tubes, bath for, copper, with extra cover	no.	1
Incubator, lead-lined, cm. 45.5 x 21.5 x 30.5	no.	1	Test tubes, thin glass, 15 cm. x 18 mm.		
Micro-burner, 1 flame	no.	1	bore	no.	300
Paper, filtering (Swedish)	qr.	1	Thermometer, 0-50° C	no.	2
Pipettes, 1-c. c	no.	2	Thermometer, 0-200° C	no.	1
Platinum wire, heavy, 10-cm	pieces.	3			

LIST OF BOOKS CONTAINED IN BERMINGHAM'S MEDICAL LIBRARY.

SET No. 1, 1882, 7 VOLUMES.

Change of Life	Tilt.
Concussion of the Spine	Erichsen.
Diseases of Modern Life	Richardson.
Diseases of the Rectum	Allingham.
Handbook of Treatment	Aitkin.
Neuralgia, etc	Anstie.
Scrofula and its Gland Diseases	Treves.

SET No. 2, 1883, 7 VOLUMES.

Diseases of the Ear	Pomeroy.
Diseases of Women, Vol. 1	Hewitt.
Diseases of Women, Vol. 2	Hewitt.
Genito-Urinary Diseases, Vol. 1	Otis.
Genito-Urinary Diseases, Vol. 2	Otis.
Impotence in the Male	Hammond.
Insanity	Spitzka.

SET No. 3, 1883 AND 1884, 7 VOLUMES.

Diseases of the Hip*	Gibney.
Excessive Venery, etc†	Howe.
Materia Medica, Vol. 1†	Nothnagel and Rossbach.
Medical Jurisprudence†	Hamilton.
Operative Surgery, Vol. 1*	Bryant.
Operative Surgery, Vol. 2*	Bryant.
Surgical Emergencies†	Von Lasser.

*1884.   †1883.

SET No. 4, 1884, 7 VOLUMES.

Diseases of the Heart	Clark.
Diseases of the Heart and Lungs	Leaming.
Favorite Prescriptions	Palmer.
Materia Medica, Vol. 2	Nothnagel and Rossback.
Materia Medica, Vol. 3	Nothnagel and Rossbach.
Medical Diagnosis	Brown.
Midwifery	Milne.

LIST OF BOOKS CONTAINED IN WOOD'S LIBRARY OF STANDARD MEDICAL AUTHORS.

BY YEARS, 1879 TO 1887, INCLUSIVE.

This volume was published in 1887 to complete the work, and is the last volume of the "Library."

45

TOOL CHEST.

CONTENTS.

1 awl, brad, and handle, 1 by ⅛ inch wide.
1 awl, brad, and handle, 1½ by ⅞ inch wide.
1 awl, brad, and handle, 2 by ⅞ inch wide.
1 awl, scratch, cast steel, 8-inch.
1 bit, auger, cast steel, ½-inch.
1 bit, auger, cast steel, ¾-inch.
1 bit, auger, cast steel, 1-inch.
1 bit, gimlet, double cut, No. 1, cast steel.
1 bit, gimlet, double cut, No. 2, cast steel.
1 bit, gimlet, double cut, No. 3, cast steel.
1 bit, screw-driver, extra cast steel, polished.
1 brace, Spofford's nickel, improved, 7-inch sweep.
1 chalk line, soft, with reel and awl complete.
1 chisel, firmer, c st steel socket, ½-inch.
1 chisel, firmer, cast steel socket, 1-inch.
1 chisel, firmer, cast steel socket, 1½-inch.
1 divider, with set screw, solid cast steel, 8-inch.
1 drawing knife, carpenter's, oval blade, 10-inch.
1 file, handsaw, with handle, 3 inches long.
1 file, handsaw, with handle, 4 inches long.
1 file, handsaw, with handle, 4½ inches long.
1 file, bastard, flat, with handle, 10 inches long.
1 gimlet, double cut, wood handle, No. 1.
1 gimlet, double cut, wood handle, No. 2.
1 gimlet, double cut, wood handle, No. 3.
1 gauge, marking, beechwood, with set screw.
1 hammer, nail, adz-eye, cast steel.
1 hatchet, shingling.

1 mallet, carpenter's, mortised handle, 5 inches long.
1 nail puller, large.
1 nail set, square, polished, solid cast steel, 4-inch.
1 nails, box of, steel wire, assorted ("Solomon Gundy").
1 nippers, plier and cutting, combined, 6-inch.
1 oiler, zinc, No. 2.
1 oilstone (Washita), 1½ lbs.
1 pinchers, carpenter's, steel jaw, 10-inch.
1 plane, fore, double iron.
1 plane, jack, double iron.
1 plane, rabbet, double iron.
1 plane, smoothing, double iron.
1 plane, hollow, No. 10.
1 plane, rounding, No. 10.
1 rasp, wood, oral, with handle, 10 inches long.
1 rule, boxwood, square joint, 8ths and 16ths, 1 inch wide, 2-foot.
1 saw, hand, 26-inch.
1 saw, panel, 16-inch.
1 saw, rip.
1 screw-driver, solid cast steel, 4-inch.
1 screw-driver, solid cast steel, 5-inch.
1 screw, hand, 8-inch.
1 screw wrench, wrought bar, 10-inch.
1 spirit level, pocket, iron top plate, japanned.
1 spokeshave, wood, 3-inch.
1 try square, rosewood, graduated, steel blade, 9-inch.
1 vise, bench, and iron.

In chest with hasp hinges, corners with angle irons, handle on each end, lock and key.

MEDICAL CHEST, U. S. ARMY, No. 1.

A list of contents is stamped on morocco pad, which is carried, reversed, under the cover of chest.

CONTENTS OF TRAY.

LEFT OF TRAY—TABLETS IN 120-C. C. BOTTLES.		
Acetanilidum	mgms.	200
Camphora et opium		
Carminative		
Catharticæ composite		
Copaibæ composite		
Ipecacuanha et opium	mgms.	324
Linimentum rubefaciens		
Magnesii sulphas, in bulk		
Mistura glycyrrhizæ comp		
Potassii bromidum	mgms.	324
Quininæ sulphas (2 bottles)	mgms.	200
Sodii bicarbonas	mgms.	324
Sodii bicarb. et menthæ pip		
Sodii salicylas	mgms.	324
And one empty bottle.		

FRONT OF TRAY—TABLETS IN 15-C. C. BOTTLES.		
Acidum arsenosum	mgm.	1
Argenti nitras fusus	grms.	15
Capsicum	mgms.	32

Cupri arsenis	mgms.	0.325
Digitalis tinctura	c.c.	0.3
Ferri composite		
Hydrargyri iodidum flavum	mgms.	10
Ergotinum	mgms.	130
Oleum tiglii	c.c.	0.006
Podophylli resina	mgms.	16
Santoninum	mgms.	32
And two empty bottles.		

BACK OF TRAY—In 235 AND 475 C. C. BOTTLES.		
Æther	c.c.	475
Alcohol	c.c.	475
Aqua ammoniæ	c.c.	235
Chloroformum	c.c.	235
Oleum ricini	c.c.	235
Oleum terebinthinæ	c.c.	235
Spiritus frumenti	c.c.	475
Spiritus vini gallici	c.c.	475
Stoppers, rubber, for above	no.	10

MEDICAL CHEST, U. S. ARMY, No. 1—Continued.

CONTENTS OF TRAY—Continued.

CENTER OF TRAY.		
Cotton	q. s.	
Envelope, small, for tablets	no.	100
Graduate, glass, 60-c. c.	no.	1
Labels for vials	no.	50
Links, split, for pack saddle	no.	4
Measure, graduated, 5-c. c.	no.	1
Ointment boxes, in nests of three	nests.	4
Pocket store	no.	1
Vials, 60-c. c.	no.	10
RIGHT OF TRAY—TABLETS IN 60-C. C. BOTTLES.		
Acidum boricum	mgms.	324
Acidum tannicum	mgms.	324
Aconiti tinctura	c. c.	0.1
Alumen	mgms.	324
Ammonii chloridi trochisci		

Antipyrinum	mgms.	324
Bismuthi subnitras	mgms.	324
Chloral	mgms.	324
Hydrarg. chl. mite cum sodio bicarb		
Hydrargyri massa	mgms.	324
Ipecacuanha	mgms.	65
Morphinæ sulphas	mgms.	8
Opium	mgms.	65
Phenacetinum	mgms.	324
Plumbi acetas	mgms.	130
Potassii chloras	mgms.	324
Potassii iodidum	mgms.	324
Salol	mgms.	324
Zinci sulphas	mgms.	324
And one empty bottle.		

CONTENTS OF DRAWERS.

DRAWER No. 1.

* HYPODERMIC TABLETS.

Apomorphinæ hydrochloras	mgms.	6
Atropinæ sulphas	mgms.	0.65
Cocainæ hydrochloras	mgms.	10
Digitalinum	mgm.	1
Morphinæ sulphas	mgms.	8
Nitroglycerinum	mgms.	0.65
Quininæ hydrochloras	mgms.	32
And one empty bottle.		

OPHTHALMIC DISCS.

Atropinæ sulphas, 0.13-mgm., 50 in box	box. 1
Physostigminæ sulphas, 0.0325-mgm., 50 in box	box. 1

MISCELLANEOUS.

Candle holder, rubber	no.	1
Corkscrew, folding	no.	1
Medicine droppers	no.	2
Pencil, indelible	no.	1
Pencil, indelible, leads for	no.	6
Pencils, camel's-hair	no.	12
Syringe, hypodermic	no.	1
Thermometer, clinical	no.	1
Tongue depressor	no.	1

DRAWER No. 2.

Bandages, suspensory	no.	5
Flannel, red	meter.	1
Jute, in 100-gm. pkgs	pkgs.	4
Syringe, rubber, self-injecting	no.	1

DRAWER No. 3.

Book, prescription	no.	1
Forceps, dressing †	no.	1
Index of Medicine (Carpenter)	copy.	1
Plaster, blistering	meter.	1
Plaster, mustard	meters.	4
Reagent case ‡	no.	1
Scissors	no.	1
Spatula	no.	1
Spoon, tea	no.	1
Stethoscope, h. r	no.	1
Syringes, p. g., in wooden case	no.	3
Syringes, p., h. r	no.	5
Tags, diagnosis, 24 in book	book.	1
Towels	no.	2

DRAWER No. 4.

Beef extract, in 100-gm. tins	tin.	1
Jute, 100-gm. pkgs	pkgs.	6

DRAWER No. 5.

Bandages, roller, assorted	no.	30
Cotton, absorbent, 100-gm. pkgs	pkgs.	4
Soap, Castile	gms.	225

DRAWER No. 6.

Candles	no.	18
Flaxseed meal	kilo.	1

DRAWER No. 7.

Cupping tins	no.	4
Gauze, plain, 1-meter pkgs	pkgs.	3
Lint, absorbent, 100-gm. pkgs	pkgs.	4
Scarificator	no.	1

* The contents of tubes of hypodermic tablets hereafter issued to replace those expended should be placed in the screw-cap bottles.

† For convenient removal of cotton from tablet bottles.

‡ Consisting of—

Acid, citric	tube	1	Sugar test powder	tube 1
Dropper, medicine	no.	1	Test tube	no. 1
Paper, litmus, blue	slips	6	Urinometer	no. 1
Potassium ferrocyanid	tube	1	With circular of directions.	

47

SURGICAL CHEST, U. S. ARMY, No. 2.

A list of contents is stamped on morocco pad, which is carried, reversed, under the cover of the chest.

CONTENTS OF TRAY.

TABLETS IN 120-C. C. BOTTLES.	
Acidum boricum_____mgms.	324
Antiseptic (2 bottles)_____	
Cathartioæ compositæ_____	
Opium_____mgms.	65
Potassii bromidum_____mgms.	324
Æther, in 500-c. c. tins_____tin.	1
Bucket, folding, canvas_____no.	1
Catheters, flexible_____no.	6
Dressing paper_____roll.	1
Felt for splints_____pieces.	2
Links, split, for pack saddle_____no.	4
Muslin_____meters.	3

TABLETS IN 235-GM. BOTTLES.	
Acidum carbolicum_____bott.	1
Chloroformum_____botts.	2
Glycerinum_____bott.	1
Opii tinctura_____bott.	1
Spiritus frumenti_____botts.	2
Stoppers, rubber, for above_____no.	10
Petrolatum_____ki'o.	½
Pocket case, aseptic_____no.	1
Pus basin_____no.	1
Razor_____no.	1
Razor strop_____no.	1
Towels_____no.	2

DRAWER No. 1.

Bandage, rubber_____no.	1	Pencil, indelible, leads for_____no.	3
Brush, nail_____no.	1	Pins, common_____paper.	1
Gauze, plain_____meters.	2	Pins, safety, assorted_____doz.	4
Goggles_____no.	2	Plaster, isinglass_____meters.	9
Iodoform sprinkler_____no.	1	Speculum for ear and nose_____no.	1
Ligature catgut, sterilized_____spools.	3	Tape_____piece.	1
Ligature silk_____gms.	15	Tape measure_____no.	1
Needles, thread, etc., in case_____case.	1	Tourniquet (Esmarch's)_____no.	1

DRAWER No. 2.

Case, tooth extracting*_____no.	1	Plaster, adhesive, 30 mm_____spool.	1
Cotton, absorbent_____pkgs.	2	Sponges, in bags_____bags.	2
Drainage tubes, rubber_____meters.	3	Syringe, fountain_____no.	1
Plaster, adhesive, 15 mm_____spools.	4		

DRAWER No. 3.

Bandages, suspensory_____no.	2	Needle, upholsterer's_____no.	1
Beef extract, in 100-gm. tins_____tin.	1	Pencil, indelible_____no.	1
Brush, shaving_____no.	1	Scissors_____no.	1
Cotton, absorbent_____pkgs.	2	Surgery, Operative, Smith's_____copy.	1
Measure, graduated, 5-c. c_____no.	1	Syringe, p., h. r_____no.	2
Medicine measuring glass_____no.	1	Tags, diagnosis, 24 in book_____book.	1
Needle, sail_____no.	1	Tool, universal_____no.	1

* This tooth-extracting case consists of—

Case, leather, rolling_____no_____1		Forceps, "half curved" root_____no_____1
Lancet, gum_____no_____1		Forceps, "lower wisdom"_____no_____1
Elevator_____no_____1		Forceps, "wisdom"_____no_____1

DRAWER No. 4.

Bandages, flannel ...	no.	4	Emergency case, complete ... no.	1
Bandages, roller ...	no.	6		

DRAWER No. 5.

Gauze, plain ... meters.	4	Lantern, small ... no.	1
Jute, in 100-gm. pkgs ... pkgs.	6	Soap, Castile ... gms.	225

DRAWER No. 6.

Bandages, roller, assorted, doz., 4.

COMMODE CHEST, No. 3.

CONTENTS.			Paper, toilet ... pkgs.	6
Bedpan, agate ware ... no.		1	Spit cup, agate ware ... no.	1
Chamber pot, agate ware ... no.		1	Urinal, agate ware ... no.	1

FIELD DESK, No. 4.

CONTENTS.

BOOKS.			Paper, blotting ... pieces q. s.	
Army Regulations ... copy.		1	Paper fasteners ... no.	12
Drill Regulations for the Hospital Corps ... copy.		1	Paper, writing, legal cap ... qr.	1
Epitome of Tripler's Manual, Greenleaf's ... copy.		1	Paper, writing, letter ... qrs.	2
Handbook for the Hospital Corps, Smart ... copy.		1	Paper, writing, note ... qr.	1
Information slip book ... copy.		1	Pencils, lead ... no.	4
Information slip book, desertions ... copy.		1	Pens, steel ... no.	12
Morning Report, Hospital Corps ... copy.		1	Penholders ... no.	2
Morning Report, sick and wounded ... copy.		1	Rubber ... piece.	1
Order and letter book ... copy.		1	Ruler ... no.	1
Register and prescription book ... copy.		1	BLANKS.	
Supply Table ... copy.		1	MEDICAL DEPARTMENT.	
Transfer book ... copy.		1		
STATIONERY.			Examination of recruits, monthly report ... no.	4
Book, blank, 8 mo ... no.		1	Hospital fund statement ... no.	4
Elastic bands, assorted ... gross.		½	Medical property, return of ... no.	2
Envelopes, official, large ... no.		12	Medical supplies, invoice of, single sheet ... no.	6
Envelopes, official, letter ... no.		50	Medical supplies, receipt for, single sheet ... no.	6
Envelopes, official, note ... no.		25	Medical supplies, special requisition for ... no.	8
Eraser, steel ... no.		1	Report of sick and wounded ... no.	12
Ink, black ... botts.		2	Report of completed cases ... no.	12
Ink, red ... bott.		1	Return of personnel, etc., H. C. ... no.	6
Inkstands ... no.		2	QUARTERMASTER'S DEPARTMENT.	
Mailing tubes ... no.		4	Clothing and equipage, quarterly return of ... no.	2
Pads, letter ... no.		1	Clothing and equipage, requisition for ... no.	4
Pads, prescription ... no.		4	Fuel, forage, and straw, requisition for ... no.	4

FIELD DESK, No. 4—Continued.

QUARTERMASTER'S DEPARTMENT—continued.		ADJUTANT-GENERAL'S DEPARTMENT.	
Invoices, abstract "E" _____no.	2	Certificates of disability_____no.	2
Receipt roll of clothing issued_____no.	2	Descriptive lists _____no.	2
Receipts, abstract "E" _____no.	2	Discharges _____no.	2
Requisitions, special (No. 48)_____no.	6	Final statements_____no.	4
Stores, quarterly return of_____no.	2	Furloughs _____no.	2
SUBSISTENCE DEPARTMENT.		Inventory of effects of deceased soldiers____no.	2
Ration returns _____no.	12	Muster rolls_____no.	8
ORDNANCE DEPARTMENT.		Outline figure cards _____no.	6
Invoices _____no.	2	Pay rolls_____no.	12
Quarterly statements _____no.	2	Physical examination of recruits, form for _no.	6
Receipts _____no.	2	Surgeon's certificate of disability for officers_no.	2

MESS CHEST, No. 5.

CONTENTS.				
Basin, wash hand, agate ware _____no.	1	Lantern, candle_____no.	1
Boilers, double, agate ware _____no.	1	Matches, in waterproof case_____boxes.	12
Bowls, soup, agate ware_____no.	6	Meat cutter, small_____no.	1
Box for salt _____no.	1	Meat dishes, agate ware_____no.	2
Box for pepper _____no.	1	Mill, coffee_____no.	1
Brush, scrubbing_____no.	1	Pan, frying, steel_____no.	1
Can openers_____no.	2	Pans, mess, agate ware _____no.	2
Cleaver_____no.	1	Pans, sauce, steel, tinned inside, with cover___no.	1
Cook book, Army _____no.	1	Plates, dinner, agate ware_____no.	6
Cups, coffee, agate ware_____no.	6	Pot, coffee, agate ware_____no.	1
Cups, large, agate ware_____no.	1	Pot, tea, agate ware_____no.	1
Dippers, agate ware_____no.	1	Rope, 6-mm_____meters.	15
Graters, nutmeg _____no.	1	Sickle _____no.	1
Gridiron_____no.	1	Spoons, basting, agate ware _____no.	1
Hatchet_____no.	1	Spoons, table _____no.	6
Kettles, steel, nested, with corers _____no.	3	Spoons, tea_____no.	6
Knife, butcher_____no.	1	Steel _____no.	1
Knife and fork, carving, of each _____no.	1	Towels, crash_____no.	6
Knife and saw, combined _____no.	1	Tray, metal, japaned_____no.	1
Knives and forks, of each _____no.	6	Tumblers, agate ware_____no.	6
Ladle, agate ware_____no.	1	Wire _____coil.	1

FOOD CHEST, No. 6.

In this chest considerable vacant space is left in order to allow latitude to each medical officer as to the exact character of the supplies he may wish to carry.

The printed plan inside the cover gives the general arrangement.

Tins labeled "corn starch," "chocolate," and "arrowroot," are included, although not mentioned in the official list of contents, as it is thought that they may contain articles of more general use.

CONTENTS.

Beef extract or an equivalent preparation.
Candles.
Condensed milk, in original cans, 4 kilos.
Soap.
Vinegar, in 1-liter wicker-covered bottles, 2 bottles.
Yeast powder, in ¼-kilo. original cans.

Tins for the following articles:
Beans.
Butter.
Coffee.
Salt and pepper.
Sugar (2 tins).
Tea.

RESERVE CHEST, No. 7.

The contents of this chest will be stated subsequently.

FOLDING FIELD FURNITURE.

A set consists of—

Chairs, arm, folding	no.	1	Table, mess, folding	no.	1
Chair, small, folding	no.	10	Tables, bedside, folding	no.	10
Cots, adjustable, folding	no.	10			

PACK SADDLE.

The new pack saddle, issued for use with the medical and surgical chests, at present consists of—

One tree, with pads and latigos.
One breast strap.
One breeching harness.
One crupper.
Two girths.
Two ropes, leather tipped.
One surcingle.
One halter and watering bridle (complete).
Two saddle blankets.
Two canvas covers for medical and surgical chests.

Four split links are carried in each medical and surgical chest for attaching them at varying heights to the pack saddle.

OUTFIT OF SCHUEHLE ICE MACHINE AS PER LATEST CONTRACT.

Ice machine, complete, Jacob Schuehle's patent, capacity 3,000 pounds in 24 hours, consists of—

1 double ammonia compressor.
1 steam engine.
1 boiler, 20-horse power, complete, with feed pump.
1 ammonia condenser.
1 $\frac{7}{10}$-inch boiler-steel freezing tank, incased in 1-inch pine flooring, with the requisite number of ice cans.
1 steam condenser, capacity sufficient to furnish in 24 hours distilled water for 3,000 pounds of ice.
1 brine pump.
1 patent oil eliminator.
1 side-feed lubricator.
300 fire brick.
Bedplate, necessary pipes, gauges, valves, connections, etc.

Anhydrous ammonia and lubricating oil sufficient to run the machine for two years.

In most cases additional or improved parts have been purchased for these machines, and this list can be considered as approximate only. The ammonia drum or cylinder is a container of the ammonia furnished by contract, and unless purchased from the ice fund does not form a part of the Schuehle machine, being returned when a fresh drum of ammonia is received. The Wood-Bailie machine, of which two are now in use, has an ammonia drum as part of the original machine. See par. 45 and Circular S. G. O., June 13, 1891.

For convenient reference the following lists are appended, although the articles are not issued by the Medical Department:

ISSUED BY THE QUARTERMASTER'S DEPARTMENT.

Ambulance.	Hatchet.	Spade.
Ambulance, harness for.	Ladder.	Stoves, heating.
Ax.	Lamps, bracket.	Tentage, etc.
Clothing, uniforms, etc.	Lamps, hanging.	Travois.
Cooking utensils.	Lockers.	Wheelbarrow.
Dippers.	Piping for ranges and stoves.	Wood saw
Flags.*	Range and fixtures.	
Gas fixtures.	Shovel.	
Hand cart.	Shelter for meteorological instruments.	

* See A. R. 1848, as amended by G. O. 83, 1880. Except guidons, these flags will rarely be issued.

ISSUED BY THE ORDNANCE DEPARTMENT.

Blanket bag.	Haversack strap.	Shotgun, reloading outfit.**
Blanket bag, shoulder straps, pair.	Knife.	Spoon.
Blanket bag, coat straps.	Knife, Hospital Corps.	Sword belt for hospital steward.
Canteen.	Knife, Hospital Corps, scabbard.	Sword-belt plate for hospital steward.
Canteen strap.	Meat can.	Sword frog for belt.
Cup, tin.	Revolver.*	Waist belt.
Fork.	Rifle, Springfield, muzzle-loading.†	Waist-belt plate.
Haversack.	Shotgun, Springfield.‡	

* Revolvers will be obtained from the Post Commander for service in an Indian country, when necessary.

† The issue of two Springfield muzzle-loading rifles to each military post for company bearers' drill is authorized. Decision Acting Secretary of War, 1888.

‡ "Upon requisition of the Post Surgeon (through the usual military channels), duly approved by the Surgeon General, the Ordnance Department will issue, for use at posts west of the Mississippi River, a shotgun, with necessary appendages and ammunition, for the use of members of the Hospital Corps." Decision Chief of Ordnance, 1889.

** The reloading outfit of the shotgun consists of the following. Expendable articles may be replaced by annual requisition upon the Chief Ordnance Officer of the Department:

Brush wiper	no	1
Canister, tin, for powder, 2-lb	no	1
Canister, tin, for powder, 5-lb	no	1
Cartridge primers	no	1,000
Cartridge shells, 20-gauge	no	50
Charger, adjustable	no	1
Cotton cloth	yd	1
Cotton waste	lbs	1¼

Drift	no	1
Funnel	no	1
Gun wads, No. 18, pink edge	no	2,000
Packing box	no	1
Powder, musket	lbs	7
Priming tool (Frankford)	no	1
Shot, No. 8	lbs	50

O

www.ingramcontent.com/pod-product-compliance
Lightning Source LLC
Chambersburg PA
CBHW022025190326
41519CB00010B/1597